D0083708

Abject Relations

Studies in Medical Anthropology

Edited by Mac Marshall

Advisory Board

William Dressler

Sue E. Estroff

Peter Guarnaccia

Alan Harwood

Craig R. Janes

Sharon Kaufman

Lynn Morgan

Catherine Panter-Brick

Stacy Leigh Pigg

Lorna Rhodes

Abject Relations

Everyday Worlds of Anorexia

LIBRARY
MILWAUKEE AREA
TECHNICAL COLLEGE
NORTH CAMPUS
5555 W. Highland Road
Mequon, WI 53092
Withdrawn
from the
MATC Library

MEGAN WARIN

RUTGERS UNIVERSITY PRESS
NEW BRUNSWICK, NEW JERSEY, AND LONDON

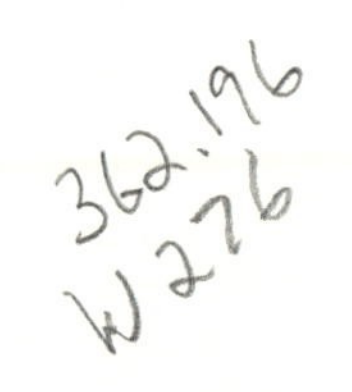

LIBRARY OF CONGRESS CATALOGING-IN-PUBLICATION DATA

Warin, Megan.
Abject relations : everyday worlds of anorexia / Megan Warin.
p. cm. — (Studies in medical anthropology)
Includes bibliographical references and index.
ISBN 978-0-8135-4689-6 (hardcover : alk. paper)
ISBN 978-0-8135-4690-2 (pbk. : alk. paper)
1. Anorexia nervosa. 2. Anorexia nervosa—Patients—Psychology.
3. Anorexia nervosa—Social aspects. I. Title.
RC552.A5W37 2009
362.196'85262—dc22

2009008099

A British Cataloging-in-Publication record for this book is available
from the British Library.

Copyright © 2010 by Megan Warin

All rights reserved

No part of this book may be reproduced or utilized in any form or by any means, electronic or mechanical, or by any information storage and retrieval system, without written permission from the publisher. Please contact Rutgers University Press, 100 Joyce Kilmer Avenue, Piscataway, NJ 08854-8099. The only exception to this prohibition is "fair use" as defined by U.S. copyright law.

Visit our Web site: http://rutgerspress.rutgers.edu

Manufactured in the United States of America

To Cameron, Freya, and Evie

CONTENTS

PREFACE

When I started the research for this book, a colleague suggested that "anorexia has been done to death." Indeed, there is much written about anorexia and it has a very firm hold in the public imagination. As a social anthropologist, however, I was dissatisfied with what I had read about anorexia. There is a strong biomedical contour to much of the literature, in which culture is compartmentalized as a culture-bound syndrome, a variable, or a risk factor, or simply seen as a context for conformity or control. While anthropologists debate the definition of "culture," in the eating-disorder field, culture is anything that is not biological, a definition that supports the fixed division between what is fact and what is constructed. Of course feminist work has importantly highlighted patriarchy, power, and gender relations as causal factors in the development of anorexia, but I was left asking these questions: Is anorexia a protest or an extreme conformity to societal ideas? Is it a cry for attention or a desire to disappear from view? Why is anorexia so difficult to treat? What do people with this diagnosis think about anorexia? It was this frustration, and an enduring interest in the anthropology of bodies, that led to this study. I knew that there was a different story to be told and that anthropology's unique approach and analysis of culture might help to unpack some of these contradictions and complexities.

Unlike behavioral/attitudinal studies and population surveys that aim to capture and configure data, an ethnographic research strategy allowed me to immerse myself in people's everyday worlds and engage with them on their own terms. I discovered what counted to people with anorexia. Long-term fieldwork provided me with very different types of knowledge simply because of its unique methodology. At first, some psychiatrists were wary of me developing close working relationships with participants, but without such connections, I could not examine the social context in which anorexia developed and flourished.

It is this ethnographic engagement with anorexia that I offer as a new contribution to the field. In 2004, eminent scholars writing for a special edition of *Culture, Medicine, and Psychiatry* on cross-cultural studies of anorexia highlighted the potential contribution of ethnographic data and social analyses to perspectives on eating disorders, and specifically asked for anthropological work to be applied to Euro-American communities where most of the research on eating disorders has been published. U.S. anthropologists O'Connor and van Esterik (2008) also call for anorexia to be demedicalized and placed within a biocultural context. This book attempts to respond to these calls by providing an alternative understanding of anorexia, one that will help make sense of the complexities of anorexia and forge new therapeutic trajectories.

ACKNOWLEDGMENTS

This book is indebted to the participants who so generously shared their time and experiences with me. It is their incredible generosity that created and sustained this project and I sincerely thank them for allowing me to share a part of their worlds.

As with any research, the ideas presented here have developed in my engagement with a wide range of other people. Unfortunately I cannot mention them all, but it is with deep gratitude that I thank those who have trained and mentored me as a social anthropologist. Deane Fergie inspired me as an undergraduate and has continued to inspire me with her intellectual wit and fortitude. Rod Lucas and Rob Barrett provided me with an apprenticeship in cultural psychiatry and introduced me to the values of ethnography and to the historical links between psychiatry, phenomenology, and anthropology. Margie Ripper honed my attention to gender relations and provided an intellectual environment where my ideas were challenged and extended. It is the superb tutelage of all these scholars that prepared me for the research on which this book is based and nurtured the process as it developed. Although these four would deny working any magic, it is their outstanding intellect and inspiration that I pay tribute to. I am honored to have worked with such eminent academics and generous people.

A great number of people assisted in making this research possible. Many health professionals welcomed me into their workplaces and gave me encouragement of all kinds. I am especially grateful to Elliot Goldner, Margaret Norman, Rolf Breyer, May McNicol, Peter Gilchrist, Charlotte Procter, Chris Freeman, Maggie Gray, Vonnie Coopman, and Cina Mastrantone.

Jon Telfer and Karen Turner read drafts of this book, and I have benefited enormously from their meticulous attention to detail, insightful comments, and encouragement at crucial moments. I also wish to thank Elspeth Probyn, Martha Macintyre, and Carole Browner for their careful reviews of drafts of this book, and their generous enthusiasm and exacting criticisms. Adi Hovav, from Rutgers University Press, has enabled this book to come to fruition, and I thank her and her colleagues for their professionalism and commitment. Bobbe Needham provided meticulous editing skills, and I am extremely grateful for this exactitude.

Others who encouraged me at crucial points along the way include John Coveney, Mandy Thomas, Fran Baum, Chilla Bulbeck, Marg Allen, Vivienne Moore, John Gray, Kay Schaffer, Catherine Panter Brick, Tessa Pollard, and Michael Carrithers.

I am grateful to all the postgraduate students and staff in the Departments of Anthropology and Social Inquiry at the University of Adelaide and University of Durham who have engaged with this work and offered intellectual stimulus in seminars, postgraduate meetings, and informal conversations (most notably the weekly morning tea in Social Inquiry). In particular, I would like to thank Nicole Moulding, Catherine Palmer, Simone Dennis, Debbi Long, Arthur Saniotis, Erez Cohen, Melissa Iocco, Lara Palombo, Pam Papadelos, Ingrid Hofmann, Emily Potter, Damon Parker, Ali Ben Kahn, Susan Oakley, Kathy Muir, Thalia Palmer, Sharon Lewis, and Colleen Solly—all of whom have skills and knowledge that have in a myriad of ways informed this work. I also wish to acknowledge the intellectual stimulation I gained from the "Eat Me! An Anthropological Examination of Food" session at the 2001 Australian Anthropological Society's annual conference at La Trobe University in Melbourne. Many thanks to the wonderful Kalissa Alexeyeff and Roberta James, and all the other panel contributors and audience members who offered critiques and suggestions.

Financial support for this project was provided by the Catherine Helen Spence Travelling Scholarship, the Karen Halley Trust, and an Australian Postgraduate Award. I thank the organizations and their administrators responsible for such vital support. A special thanks to Peter and Karin Wood, local knowledge brokers of Catherine Helen Spence's early years, in Melrose, Scotland.

And finally, I wish to thank my family. I am indebted to Joan's and Jack's belief in the value of education and fostering a love of learning. To my partner, Cameron, I am indebted for unstinting encouragement and confidence in me to achieve on so many levels. And to Freya and Evie, thank you for allowing me to take the time to write.

I am grateful to the publishers of the following articles, who granted permission to reproduce parts of them for this book:

Warin, M. 2006. "Reconfiguring Relatedness in Anorexia." *Anthropology and Medicine* 13(1): 41–54.

Warin, M. 2005. "Transformations of Intimacy and Sociality: Bedrooms in Public Institutions." *Body and Society* 11(3): 97–113.

Warin, M. 2004. "Primitivising Anorexia: The Irresistible Spectacle of Not Eating." *Australian Journal of Anthropology* 15(1): 95–104.

Warin, M. 2003. "Be-coming Clean: The Logic of Hygiene in Anorexia." *SITES: A Journal of Social Anthropology and Cultural Studies* 1(1): 109–132.

Warin, M. 2003. "Miasmatic Calories and Saturating Fats: Fear of Contamination in Anorexia." *Culture, Medicine, and Psychiatry* 27: 77–93.

Abject Relations

1

Introduction

The air of anticipation among the young women in this suburban Vancouver community house had been building all week, simmering in summer conversations on the veranda, then spilling over into therapy sessions with staff. As a group, the women told me about the nameless "underweight woman" who was coming to stay with them for a brief period. Her emaciated state was their central concern, for all the women in this program had gained weight through a recovery program and were still adjusting to their new embodied presence. A few days later this anonymous person had a name. "Josie will sabotage all our hard work just by being here," Sophie complained to the nurses.[1]

Although she was expected to arrive in time for the evening dinner, Josie had been held up at the hospital by appointments with doctors. This delay only added to the suspense. She must be "really sick," the residents said. Josie arrived just as the eight women on the recovery program were sitting down to debrief after their shared evening meal (her timing could not have been better). When everyone gathered in the lounge and took up their usual seats, Josie was already perched in the middle of a large sofa, the center of attention. The women sneaked glances to assess her diminutive frame, the large water bottle placed between her knees, the prominent veins in her arms and legs, her waxy skin and protruding cheekbones. Despite her cadaverlike appearance, Josie's demeanor did not communicate sickness, weakness, or fatigue. She sat upright, her head high, her strong voice and direct eye contact reflecting the power of the unease she had created. She held center stage, and the other women (including me) were silent, drawn to her presence.

This scene captures the central ethnographic and analytic themes that underpin this book: relatedness and abjection. Josie knew that she held a position of distinction in the group. She embodied what many longed to return to—pure anorexia, a clean state of being untainted by the polluting aspects of food, one's body, and relationships. She firmly belonged to what some referred to as "the anorexia club," an elite and secretive group that strategically mobilized the term "anorexia" for its own purposes. Josie was not disempowered by the label of disorder. On the contrary, it afforded her a symbolic power that the others had relinquished. Her level of sickness only served to heighten her position of power within the room. By entering into a contract of recovery, the eight women no longer belonged to anorexia; they had cut the cord and sullied themselves by imbibing food. Several told me afterward that returning to normal health disgusted them, and the desire to move back to anorexia—to be clean, empty, and pure—was something with which they constantly struggled.

This book is an ethnographic study of people's everyday experiences of anorexia. As a social anthropologist I am trained to question, unsettle, and find meaning in the ordinary and extraordinary practices of everyday lives, and then seek to make sense of these within broader sociocultural frameworks. In doing so, this work unpacks common understandings that have fixed anorexia as the epitome of a Western obsession with individualism, self-control, and autonomy and offers an alternative understanding. Through intensive participant observation I came to know a different logic of anorexia, one that deals with the shifting (and contradictory) forces of power, disgust, and desire. These forces do not unfold along a linear trajectory but are in constant motion, reflecting the back-and-forth strategies of making and remaking, and of connecting and disconnecting with people. This motion is primarily concerned with relatedness—relating to oneself, to others, and to the world. This book is thus concerned with what happens to people when they have a diagnosis of anorexia, and how they get along in the world.

In anthropology relatedness has traditionally been associated with kinship studies of family connections, arrangements, and obligations that were initially assumed to be grounded in the natural, biological facts of sexual procreation. A key figure in shifting these formalist traditions was Schneider (1968/1980, 1984), who in his first work argued that American kinship was a cultural system that operated through symbolic logic. Schneider suggested that sexual reproduction was a core symbol of a kinship system that comprised two distinct models of "relationship as natural substance [symbolized in idioms of blood] and relationship as code for conduct [what people do and say they do]" (1980, 29). In his 1984 book, which encompassed a commentary on his first work, *American Kinship*, he argued that the centrality of sexual procreation to anthropological models of kinship was deeply flawed due to its focus on the cultural specificity of assumed universal, natural facts (see also Needham 1971).

While in *Abject Relations* I do not dwell on contemporary debates about kinship studies, I raise Schneider's pathbreaking work to demonstrate its importance in broadening the conceptualization of relatedness.[2] Recent interest in kinship studies has questioned his problematic and at times contradictory dichotomy of the social and biological (Carsten 2000a, b, 2004; Franklin 1997, 2003). "Relatedness," as Edwards and Strathern comment, "was never one thing, and definitely never either a matter of social or biological connection alone" (2000, 162). Edwards argues elsewhere that the concept of relatedness extends beyond the presence of natural and shared substance (for example, blood or genes) and can include notions of connectedness "with or without a genetic link" (1993, 45; 2000). Relatedness is thus not simply about the separate domains of biology or the social but includes the intersections between them and beyond them.

It is in this wider focus of relatedness that I situate the arguments of this book. I argue that concepts and practices of relatedness are composed not just of ties created by procreation and familial/social obligation but of multiple elements: the everyday exchanging and sharing of food and substances, living together, domestic arrangements, places, memories, emotions, and relationships (including sexual)—"elements which are themselves not necessarily bounded entities but may overflow or contain parts of each other or take new forms" (Carsten 2000a, 34). Relatedness "permeates all domains of social life" (Edwards 2000, 27). While Holy cautions that such a general characterization of relatedness renders it in danger of "becoming analytically vacuous" (1996, 168), such broadening is required to prize relatedness away from the privileged and arbitrary distinctions of biology and culture and move it toward the everyday acts that comprise relatedness.

Ernst refers to these elements or components of relatedness as "*relations of relationships*, not relations of individuals" (Ernst 1990, 111, emphasis in original). This is an important distinction, as the analytic and folk terms that are often used interchangeably to denote idioms of relatedness ("relationships," "relatives," "relations," and "relational") are in effect differing parts of the conceptualization of relatedness. As I use it, relatedness is a multilayered continuum "comprising everything from the most formal relations of descent to the least formal relations of, say, secret friendships" (Stafford 2000, 53).

Rather than positioning anorexia and other eating disorders within a framework of individual pathology, I argue that relatedness, in all its forms, is central to people's practices and experiences of anorexia. Practices that are taken for granted as creating and sustaining relatedness—from the everyday practices of commensality to the capacity to have children—were consistently viewed negatively by participants with a diagnosis of anorexia. These practices were regarded as dirty and disgusting and feared for their threatening, yet desired, potentialities.

Negating consensual avenues of relatedness did not leave these people in a void. On the contrary, they created new meanings and experiences of being related. New forms of relatedness included concealment of anorexic practices (from family, medical staff, and friends), secrecy and competitiveness with other in-patients, friendships forged through sharing a common diagnosis, and the personification of anorexia as a friend, an abusive lover, a parent, a child, the devil in disguise, or an enemy. Some people even gave anorexia a name like Ana or Ed (the former a shortened version of anorexia and the latter an acronym of "eating disorder"). Individually and collectively, people entered into a relationship with anorexia that in turn tempered their relationship with their everyday worlds.

Central to these processual movements of relatedness were ambiguous experiences. The very term "anorexia," which literally means lack of desire, loss of appetite, or both (Peters 1995, 63), is erroneous, for a person with this diagnosis often stands in an ambiguous relationship with food, that is, "obsessed with it, she similarly regards it as an object of desire and disgust" (Celermajer 1987, 65). Participants in this study simultaneously experienced pleasure and disgust, were empowered and disempowered, felt safe yet constantly threatened, were both pure and dirty, and when sickest felt at their best. Anorexia was a constant process of becoming and unbecoming, of having a life by moving toward death.

In many ways, these experiences of relatedness have remarkable resonances with what the philosopher Julia Kristeva outlines in her theory of horror, which she terms "abjection." Located in the physical immediacy of bodies, abjection is a psychoanalytic/literary model that Kristeva uses to explain the process of self-individuation in the early years of life. Kristeva suggests that in order for a child to attain identity and a place within the symbolic order, it must separate from the "nourishing and murderous" maternal body and recognize its own bodily boundaries and limits (1982, 54). This, Kristeva argues, is a process that occurs on the threshold of acquiring language, for it is when the child learns the language associated with the clean and proper body that subjectivity is possible. By disavowing aspects of corporeality, especially those which threaten bodily boundaries—the improper, dirty, and disorderly—the child learns to mark off the self and claim the body as its own.

While the word "abject" literally means to cast off, away, or out, abjection is defined in relationship to desire. It "beseeches, worries and fascinates desire" (Kristeva 1982, 1) and is endured because of this relationship (Fuery 1995, 94). Kristeva identifies three broad forms of abjection: in relation to food and bodily incorporation; toward bodily waste; and toward the signs of sexual difference. Substances like spit, food, feces, and vomit are abject for they "disturb identity, system, order; . . . [they do] not respect borders, positions and rules; . . . [they are] in between, ambiguous, composite." As "imaginary uncanniness and real threat," what is abject must be rejected and cast out; otherwise it "ends up engulfing us" (4). As neither subject nor object, the abject is "closely bound up with questions of identity, boundary crossing, exile and displacement" (Smith 1998, 29).

While this book does not rely on Kristeva's psychoanalytic framework, it does extend her concept of abjection and ground it ethnographically. In arguing for a critical application of Kristeva's theory, I demonstrate that one cannot write about abjection without considering relatedness. Relatedness is at the very core of abjection, for, in being cast out, one moves away from relationships with people, oneself, and objects and creates a different kind of relatedness. Abjection, as I use it, moves beyond Kristeva's location of it in the imaginary, psyche, and language to the everyday practices and terms of sociality. By bringing the concepts of relatedness and abjection together into the analytical arena, this book raises new questions and new perspectives concerning not only anorexia, but also the lives of those who are given this diagnosis.

This book thus tracks the multiple dimensions of relatedness and abjection through people's experiences of anorexia. It explores what was considered abject (objects, spaces, and bodies); the embodied, visceral responses to this (simultaneous horror and fascination); and the practices by which people desired, cast out, and removed the abject. Things considered abject, including fats, bodily processes, public spaces, and relationships, were distanced, negated, cleansed, and purged in an attempt to remove their threat. While clinicians saw these practices as symptomatic of a diagnosis of anorexia nervosa, those who practiced them understood them as entitlements to anorexia, a process interwoven with revulsion and desire.

Through this ethnography, anorexia becomes a vehicle for extending not only the analytic concept of abjection, but also the notion of relatedness. Anthropological concepts of relatedness have not been addressed in any of the writings on anorexia, despite that literature being replete with negative connotations of sociality such as withdrawal, regression, lying, hidden behaviors, and toxic families (in the forms of obsessive mothers and absent fathers). Cross-cultural literature clearly demonstrates the usefulness of examining food in terms of relatedness. Becker, for example, in exploring embodied experiences in Fiji, highlights the "relational matrix" of self, body, food, kin, and community relations that underpin the oceanic ethos of social relatedness (1995, 5). Alexeyeff (2004) similarly notes how the exchange of foods among Cook Island women is very much part of a continuous and dynamic process of relatedness. Relatedness is also central to people's experiences of anorexia, yet it has been overlooked in discourses of individualism, or what Lester calls "pathologies of control" (2007, 377). Similarly, with the exception of Reineke's 1997 *Sacrificed Lives* (which discusses abjection, anorexia, and medieval women mystics within Kristeva's psychoanalytic terms), an extended and ethnographically informed theory of abjection has not been central to any exploration of anorexia.

The perpetual movement by participants in this ethnography (of their desires, connections, and ruptures) highlights the ways in which relatedness and abjection move and transform across apparently divided epistemological fields. Just as relatedness is not exclusively biological or social, abjection is not located only within or outside the individual. To challenge and question these concepts (the enduring anthropological endeavor), this book proposes that experiences of anorexia continually cross the divides that are central to abjection and relatedness, shifting from one realm to another. It is by way of these movements, and the intersections between them, that anorexia, relatedness, and abjection are experienced.

The Study: Participants and Places

I conducted the fieldwork on which this book is based in Vancouver, British Columbia; Edinburgh, Scotland; and Adelaide, South Australia in the late 1990s and early 2000. As ethnographic approaches are concerned with gathering detailed information about people's everyday lives and the meaning (not the outcome) of things, the number of people involved is much smaller than that in larger, quantitative studies. This research deals with forty-four women and three men ranging in age from fourteen to fifty-five.[3] They came from struggling farming backgrounds, migrant families, and professional families. Their residences varied from inner-city rental apartments, country homes, and housing estates to opulent mansions in leafy suburbs. Although the participants were Anglo-Celtic, they often spoke of connections and disconnections with related family homelands: Greece, Croatia, Estonia, the United Kingdom, and Germany. Occupations ranged from high school and university students (law, medicine, psychology) to people in teaching, nursing, general practice, acting, and sales assisting in retail shops. Several who were too unwell to work were surviving on financial assistance from government agencies.

While more than a third of these people lived alone, 52 percent lived with family (parents, partners, or children). This group comprised not only those who were married (five) and had children (six) but also the youngest participants of this research, thirteen of whom were under the age of twenty-three. Many of these were studying and were financially dependent on their parents. Six of them lived in share accommodation with friends, most of these studying at university. The most striking aspect of people's living arrangements was the absence of sexual relationships.[4] More than 70 percent were single and not engaged in any form of intimacy at the time of my fieldwork. In terms of relatedness, this is significant, for several described the difficulty of having other and intimate relationships while "you were having a relationship with anorexia." As Maddy, now recovered, said: "The place where anorexia is, it's a very narrow space, and there is little room for anything else."

In attempting to understand anorexia I tried to expose myself to as many of people's experiences as possible, through what Stoller calls "an assortment of ingredients—dialogue, description, metaphor, metonymy, synecdoche, irony, smells, sights and sounds" (1989, 32). This often meant accompanying people through cycles of treatment—into hospitals, on visits to treatment centers, to meetings with psychiatrists and nursing staff—and back to their own homes and everyday lives. We met in cafés, parks, and pubs, went grocery and clothes shopping, and spent hours sitting in kitchens, lounge rooms, and on bedroom floors. I thus spent time not only with those who had a diagnosis of anorexia, but also with health professionals, community and volunteer workers, health administrators, and participants' family members, neighbours, and friends. Although treatment spaces are an important part of participants' experiences, these did not define their social worlds and are not the central focus of this book. It is the comprehensive nature of fieldwork that distinguishes this book from all other writing on anorexia, an ethnographic analysis that incorporates and extends beyond an institutional and discursive framing.

Meetings were initially arranged through clinicians and community nurses, who acted as gatekeepers to a psychiatric community of eating-disorder patients. The term "community" is a misnomer, for there was no one place where people with anorexia lived together for a lengthy period of time. I did, however, have the opportunity to do fieldwork in a community treatment house where residents lived for up to four months. Most of the time, though, encounters were one to one, reflecting the isolated lives that many participants led.

While I do not claim to represent the plurality of people's experiences and their continually changing and contingent nature, I have sought to elucidate the common threads of what people experience as anorexia. Although different people had different names for anorexia, throughout this book I refer to it as anorexia, as this is the diagnosis that each was given, a label that profoundly affected their lives.[5] I recognize the desire of many to write this term out of existence (Eckermann 1994; Malson 1998, 144; Pembroke 1993), but I could not ignore the symbolic power attached to it and the strategies used to mobilize its worth. This is not to suggest that the label existed independently as a clinical entity, or that it was necessarily taken as a given (it was, at certain times, denied), but rather to point to the ways in which anorexia was mobilized and transformed by participants. Anorexia was more than a medical diagnosis; it was, among many things, an empowering state of being, a friend, an enemy, and a way of life.

In many ways I have always had a much clearer sense of what this book would not be about, and it was this steering away that directed the course of this ethnography. It is important for me to briefly articulate my differences and dissatisfaction with taken-for-granted assumptions concerning anorexia, for they provided a springboard for my analytic and ethnographic focus.

The Spectacle of Thinness

It is hard to disentangle the myriad assumptions that circulate around anorexia. It has, in the words of Appadurai, its own "social life" (1986). These assumptions have a strong hold in the public imagining of this disorder, and it seems as if everyone has some familiarity with and hence an opinion on the topic.[6] Throughout this research I have listened to and read a plethora of interpretations of anorexia: a regression to childhood; an inability to deal with adulthood; an issue of control and resistance against a universal backdrop of female subordination; a genetic predisposition; a biological dysfunction; the fault of the media promulgating images of thin models as the ideal body type; a result of toxic families; and even, as the family friend of one participant suggested, "the devil's work."[7]

Despite the differing frameworks (of feminism, medicine, psychology, history, and religion), there were common taken-for-granted representations that underpinned and limited each analysis. Each viewed the person who self-starved or who had a diagnosis of anorexia as striving toward the attainment of thinness. It was the thin body that was the focus of attention, the marker of illness or of succumbing to patriarchal ideals.[8] The thin body was the extreme body, and one that provided simultaneous horror and fascination in popular imaginings. Visual representations of this body play into the ways in which thin bodies inhabit limited space—the front cover of Naomi Wolf's *Beauty Myth* (1990) depicts a bandaged and silenced naked woman holding an orange and contorted underneath a small wooden table. Other media images have women standing sideways against blank walls, emphasizing their jutting hips and frail postures (these are often accompanied by before-and-after photographs).

Focusing on thinness creates a number of problems. It is first a privileging of the visual, of the outsider's, the colonizer's, gaze. I am reminded of Franz Kafka's 1922 short story *A Hunger Artist*, which chronicles a form of paid entertainment that was popular in traveling carnivals around the turn of the nineteenth century in Europe. In a cage spread with straw, the male hunger artist publicly fasted for forty days and nights. Permanent guards (usually butchers) watched the hunger artist day and night, "in case he should have some secret recourse to nourishment." "Children," Kafka wrote, "stood open mouthed, holding each other's hands for greater security, marvelling at him as he sat there pallid in tights, with his ribs sticking out so prominently, . . . [sometimes] stretching an arm through the bars so that one might feel how thin it was" (Kafka 1992, 268). As Gooldin (2003) notes in her account of these hunger artists, the spectacle of fasting was a particularly significant aspect of the Victorian fasting women phenomenon.

There is no doubt that thinness associated with anorexia holds fascination. It is, as the description of Josie in the opening paragraphs of this chapter attests, a spectacular end product. Many media articles use the same enticement of spectacle, with shocking color images of young women's emaciated bodies, often semi-naked. People dying of cancer are rarely represented in the same exhibitionist manner.[9] A male journalist contacted the eating-disorder association I volunteered at, wanting to interview a young woman with anorexia, and requested a "really skinny one" for the story. Focusing solely on this visual spectacle of anorexia continues to position and reproduce the female body as public, as an object to be examined, beholden and always visible. Anorexia is reduced to a carnivalesque image that is represented by femaleness, thinness, illness, horror, fascination, and death. In the wake of reflexive anthropology, I was acutely aware of not reproducing the exoticism associated with representations of anorexia.[10] Moreover, as I discuss in the conclusion of this book, these representations were too simplistic and did not allow for an understanding of anorexia that included the complexities of gendered, embodied experiences, of the power at work, or of the sense of distinction that came from such a posturing.

During my fieldwork I quickly learned to discard thinness as the definitive bodily marker of anorexia. Thinness denotes a static and fixed occupation of space and time. Most participants were not spectacularly thin, and the few who were did not remain so. Participants were continually moving through a different stage of anorexia each time we met, from being newly diagnosed, to weight gain programs, toward recovery, and in many cases, back to hospitals (including intensive care units). Rita, who became a central informant, made light of the fact that people with anorexia are not always thin. When we arranged to meet for the first time, she joked on the phone that she would be "the fat one" standing by her white car in the car park outside a public garden. I wasn't sure at the time if she was being facetious, and indeed when we met she was not the stereotypical thin anorexic. Rita had experienced both anorexia and bulimia for most of her adult life, and her weight had fluctuated dramatically. My interest though was not in her weight, but rather in her experiences of anorexia, experiences that were embodied, corporeal, felt and sensed. Her body weight was not a prerequisite to her sharing her memories, grief, and life. Her experiences of embodiment were.

Discursive Approaches

Besides discarding thinness as definitive of anorexia, the second point of departure that this research took was created by my desire not to reproduce the many discourse-orientated approaches to eating disorders. Within the vast body of literature that deals with eating disorders there is one poststructuralist thinker who stands out. Michel Foucault's theory of discourse has been highly influential and productive in this literature because it provides a double critique of medicine and, by extension, of patriarchy.[11] Writers including Bartky (1988), Bordo (1988, 1989, 1990), Eckermann (1994, 1997), Hepworth (1999), Malson (1998), Robertson (1992), Tait (1992), and Turner (1984, 1987) have drawn on Foucault's work in some measure to throw light on "the complex network of disciplinary systems and prescriptive technologies through which power operates" (Diamond and Quinby 1988, xi). Both Bordo and Bartky argue regarding self-starvation that constructions of femininity, and a preoccupation with diets/exercise, have actually constituted these disorders. Feminist literature's critique and deconstruction of femininity has suggested that powerful patriarchal discourses construct images of femininity that are contradictory, and that anorexia is a way of simultaneously resisting and complying with these ideals.

One of the ways in which patriarchal power operates, it is argued, is through the media and the dissemination of such contradictory images of femininity. Even writers like Wolf who do not directly draw upon Foucault's insights point to the ubiquitous images of thinness, beauty, and power that fill the pages of women's magazines, newspapers, films, and television screens. Wolf argues that these images have created a beauty myth that has been "masterfully orchestrated" to coerce and silence women. She views this myth as "a direct solution to the dangers posed by the women's movement and economic and reproductive freedom. Dieting is the most potent political sedative in women's history; a quietly mad population is a tractable one" (1990, 187).

Theorists with a Foucauldian perspective have offered some quite convincing explanations of anorexia itself, but, like Wolf, have tended to "read the anorexic body" as a metaphor for the social body—as Bordo's title explicitly states, a "crystallization of culture" (1988). In criticizing this approach, Bray (1994, 1996) refers to anorexia as a "reading disorder," building on the common assumption that anorexia is a pathology brought about by women's uncritical consumption of media images of thin femininity (1996, 413; see also Celermajer 1987; Gooldin 2008).[12] The anorexic body of these analyses, which in many ways reproduce the docile body that Foucault articulated, is a text on which cultural values are inscribed, etched, and written.[13] Power relations "have an immediate hold on it; they invest it, mark it, train it, torture it, force it to carry out tasks, to perform ceremonies, to emit signs" (Foucault 1977, 25). The particular use of Foucault's discourse has rendered the gendered body malleable, one that "locates the generative forces outside the immediate, lived reality of the lifeworld" (Jackson 1996, 21; see also McNay 1999).

This passivity of the body is in part a result of the way in which these writers locate discourse and its operations of power and knowledge solely in specific institutional practices—in hegemonic and dualist structures that allow little space for agency, embodiment, and the everyday. This is in spite of the theoretical shift in Foucault's own understanding of power from institutions to the self.[14] Turner, for example, demonstrates this hegemony at work: "Anorexia is . . . a symbolic struggle against forms of authority [patriarchy, family, and medicine] and an attempt to solve the contradictions of the female self, fractured by the dichotomies of reason and desire, public and private, body and self, nature and culture" (1984, 201).

In this formulation, women with anorexia not only are struggling against the oppression of male domination (which is located in a hegemonic discourse) but also are attempting to reconcile the embodiment of Cartesian ideology (again located in a hegemonic discourse) that is said to fracture all women. Despite the rhetoric of power acting in a diffuse manner, "women" (the use of the generic itself being problematic) are fundamentally caught in a web of discursively produced hierarchical positions in which they are always dominated and disadvantaged (see also Hall 1996, 12; McNay 1994).[15] McNay argues that Foucault "steps too easily from describing disciplinary power as a tendency within modern forms of social control, to positing disciplinary power as a fully installed monolithic force which saturates all social relations (1994, 104). Power, then, is always a form of domination, for in Foucault's theory, discourses "discipline" the body through a "multiplicity of minor processes of domination" (Foucault 1977, 138).

While not denying the use of power within medicine or the profound influences of Foucault's work, such an explanation cannot account for the transformative, empowering, and ambiguous experiences of anorexia—in short, for the very centrality of relatedness.[16] In my fieldwork I observed the multiple ways in which those with this diagnosis strategically deployed power.[17] Power was used quite differently from Turner's Foucauldian account. It was not a force either yielded to or coercive. In fact, it was a force taken and transformed into a productive embodied state. The power associated with anorexia was exemplified by Josie, whose extreme thinness was, to those recovering from anorexia, a mark of distinction, a state of purity, and a sign of belonging to an elite group.

In my fieldwork it was clear that the powers at play were not simply between doctors and patients; they were far more complex than allowed for in a static theory of domination. Within the collective of anorexia, for example, there were constant struggles for hierarchical positions of purity—to be the best anorexic. Similarly, in various institutions, therapists and psychiatrists vied over who had the authority to speak about anorexia, and the best way to treat anorexia was a highly contentious issue. In Pierre Bourdieu's terms, anorexia was situated and practiced in a "field," a relational social space defined by a dynamic configuration and positioning of people and structures.

In using Bourdieu's concept of field, the centrality of agency comes into play, an integral but overlooked part of social discourse. "Individuals," as Bourdieu comments "exist as agents—and not as biological individuals, actors or subjects—who are socially constituted as active and acting in the field under consideration by the fact that they possess the necessary properties to be effective, to produce effects, in this field" (Bourdieu and Wacquant 1992, 107).

On a similar note, Judith Butler in *Gender Trouble* points out that while identity is constructed, it does not follow that identity is therefore fully determined by this construction—such an argument would deny the possibility of agency.[18] "Construction is not opposed to agency," Butler writes, "it is the necessary scene of agency, the very terms in which agency is articulated and becomes culturally intelligible" (1990, 147).

While it is clearly important "to trace the discourses and practices of medicine and to demonstrate shifts as well as continuities over time," it is equally important to "allow for lived experience, for the phenomenology of the body. Bodies may be surrounded by and perceived through discourses, but they are irreducible to discourse. The body needs to be grasped as an actual material phenomenon which is both affected by and affects knowledge and society" (Lupton 1997, 103; Shilling 1991, 664).

Discourses, as Weedon points out, "exist both in written and oral forms and in the social practices of everyday life," yet the everyday has been remarkably absent in writings on anorexia (1987, 111). As the medical sociologist Eckermann points out in her discussion of eating disorders: "It could be argued that many researchers, whether writing from a feminist perspective or not, are culpable of invoking the family and the mass media as scapegoats for what might be a process more deeply embedded in our social existence than we have so far been able to fathom. It would seem that in the move from individualized and medicalized explanatory frameworks to those more socially orientated, major areas of social existence have been ignored. This process is exacerbated by insistence on distinct historical epochs with distinct sets of discourses" (1994, 92).

Ethnographic fieldwork is centrally positioned to address these lacunae. Through a range of fieldwork methodologies, ethnographers build and sustain (often long-term) relationships with participants in order to learn firsthand about their everyday worlds. Surprisingly, there are few detailed ethnographic studies of people with anorexia (see Gooldin 2008; Gremillion 1996, 2003; Lester 2007); others that claim to be ethnographic rely on interview data (and often one-time interviews). The value of spending time with people and doing intense participant observation is that we learn there is often a vast gap between what people say they do and what they actually do in their everyday lives.

The more I attuned myself to how people with anorexia conceptualized relatedness, rather than framing them within already defined discursive positionings, the more creative and dynamic were the intersections I learned from. Food was experienced as dirty and contaminating: there were practices to avoid fats being absorbed into the skin, and some participants covered their noses and mouths to avoid smells sneaking into their bodies. Food had the potential to transgress boundaries and was considered contaminating and dirty. To touch or eat food (and fats in particular) was to be avoided at all costs.

Participants repeatedly told me, however, that anorexia was not simply about food. Nor was it solely concerned with the consumption of media images. The media was often said to be a red herring. "Anorexia," one woman explained, "is way too focused on the media. People think eating disorders are solely based on body image that is warped by the media and it's all about body size; . . . it has to do with that, but it's only a small piece of the pie so to speak—using a food metaphor." According to this participant, and many others, anorexia was concerned with relatedness, with "coming into family problems, coming into relationship problems, coming into big fears." Relatedness was intensely problematic and was renegotiated through anorexic practices.

Embodied Practices

Even though I conducted a large proportion of my fieldwork in my hometown, I could never assume a shared world with those who had anorexia. I sought, however, to come closer to understanding the nature of their transformative, contradictory, and contingent experiences. My principal means of working out these understandings relied on dialogue and observation of embodied practices, what Desjarlais refers to as "a phenomenology of embodied aesthetics" (1992, 66). With participants, I shared in conversations of informal knowledge, conducted open-ended interviews, explored lyrics to songs, delved into autobiographical writings, spoke of the meanings of artworks (often their own), and examined the ways in which anorexia was represented in the media.[19] I also observed and listened to how experiences of anorexia were represented in the medical domain, attending formal presentations of cases at hospital ward rounds and, when given permission by participants, reading their confidential hospital records.

Experiences were conveyed not only through words; they were simultaneously embodied and performed. As I detail in chapter 2, I observed the ways in which arms and legs were held close to the body, limbs often moved as if exercising, and faces and bodies contorted at the suggestion of certain foods. Sophie quickly placed her hand over her stomach when it loudly rumbled and apologized for her "stomach's intrusion." We paused to consider her response and why the internal sounds of the body were considered embarrassing and must be hidden. It was by sharing spoken and gestured language (and silences and embarrassed laughs) that participants and I were able to come to a communal plane on which to understand experiences of anorexia, however partial our connection (see also Clifford and Marcus 1986; Haraway 1988; Lucas 1999; M. Strathern 1991). As Tsing reiterates: "The knowledge of an author, like that of the people about whom he or she writes, is always partial, situated, and perspectivistic" (1993, 14–15).

It was this mixture of language and experience, rather than separation, that I aimed for. Language, like experience, is spoken and gestured, held in memories, and completely contingent. The separation between semiotics and phenomenology, language and experience, and representation and being in the world is somewhat false, for language (spoken and gestured) gives access to a world of experience and simultaneously does not wholly constitute experience (sensory experiences, for example, are not circumscribed by language).[20] As Jackson states: "It is difficult to draw a line between inherited cultural knowledge and personal experience" (1996, 42). He argues that the phenomenological method aims for verisimilitude, placing primary experience and secondary elaboration (in the form of language) on the same footing. Csordas similarly argues that "the notion that language is itself a modality of being-in-the-world . . . is perhaps best captured in Heidegger's notion that language not only represents or refers, but 'discloses our being-in-the-world' " (1994, 11).[21]

In pointing to the unnecessary opposition of philosophical viewpoints (rather than the perpetual movement between them), these writers are highlighting the concept of embodiment, which has been central to all of Bourdieu's writings. It was pervasive Cartesian dichotomies, such as the one that posits representation as opposite to experience, that inspired Bourdieu to formulate his theories of habitus, capital, and field as a way of bridging the divisiveness of structuralist and objectivist arguments. What bridges these dichotomies is the body. For Bourdieu, embodiment is the principal way in which structures are internalized, practiced, transformed, and reproduced—this is Bourdieu's logic of practice, the habitus. Embodiment for Bourdieu is thus not concerned simply with phenomenology or the internalization of structures, but also with the dialectical relationship between the gendered body and space, a dialectics of structure and practice.[22] As I discuss in chapter 2,

Bourdieu's theories are thus more applicable to the arguments in this book than is Foucault's theory of power, for they explore the relational, generative, and potentially ambiguous possibilities of human action.

Outline of the Book

In her ethnography of kinship, *The Heat of the Hearth*, Carsten deliberates as to how she will describe the Malay houses that were central to her fieldwork in Langkawi. She could begin, she writes, by describing the different aspects of housing, "the appearance of the houses outside and in, their structure, design, and furnishing, the division of space within them. . . . These would all be legitimate beginnings to a story which—like all anthropological stories—has no beginning because everything connects with everything else" (1997, 33).

The concept that "everything connects with everything else" is similarly applicable to this book. To begin arbitrarily with the concept of food, one is led into numerous, overlapping fields: "Food moves all the time; . . . it leads us into other areas, . . . it spills into every aspect of life, . . . it constantly shifts registers: from the sacred to the everyday, from metaphor to materiality, it is the most common and elusive of matters" (Probyn 1999, 217).[23] The notion that food moves, connects and disconnects links directly into a central trope of this book, that of movement. Movement underpins the methodology, ethnography, and analysis.

Chapter 2 of this book explores the places in which my fieldwork unfolded. Participants moved back and forth between what Parr and Philo refer to as a "mishmash of sites" (1995, 211). These fields, multiple and overlapping, included various sites of treatment, domestic homes, and public spaces, as well as the public imagining and representations of this phenomenon.

The methodological planning and enactment of multisited fieldwork had direct implications for the theoretical underpinnings of this book, for the multiple sites in which my fieldwork occurred were analogous to the multiple fields of knowledges and representations in which people (including health professionals and those with a diagnosis of anorexia) struggled for legitimacy and authority. Drawing on Bourdieu's notion of field and related concepts of habitus and symbolic capital, this chapter connects methodology to analysis, as both seek to elucidate the underlying and invisible relations in and among social spaces.

A central question at this point might be, How does an anthropologist do fieldwork with a group of people for whom sociality and relatedness is problematic? considering that these are essential to any fieldwork situation (see Rabinow 1977, 155). Chapter 3, "Knowing through the Body," explores how I established and maintained relationships among a group of people with whom I did not share common taken-for-granted assumptions and experiences. One of the ways I engaged with them was by taking their cues of sociality as a guide. We rarely ate together; some meetings were called to a halt by participants, some were awkward, and some participants allowed me to enter their worlds based on the premise that I did not threaten them by asking they share commensality with me.

Part of this discussion enters into the debates concerning doing fieldwork at home, in places that are familiar to the ethnographer. The privileging of geographical space, of home as comfortable, near, and familiar, is in itself a construct that I question. One does not need to be spatially distant to experience strangeness, and strangeness and familiarity can operate simultaneously. It was, for example, through my own profound transformation when I was in the field—pregnancy—that the seemingly disparate experiences of strangeness and distance were collapsed. It was also via these transformations that ethnographic analogy was made between my participants and myself. Through our changing and heightened embodied sensations, we were able to find some common ground in what Jackson calls interexperience, an analogous space in which we explored the shifting embodied states of bodily dwelling.

Chapter 4 turns to a different kind of relatedness, that of desire toward and distancing from this thing called anorexia. Here I introduce a term coined by Battaglia—"agency play"—a concept that, akin to Bourdieu's notion of play and struggle, explores the various identities and agencies that people with anorexia use and discard according to differing sites. Concealment and revelation are central to these plays of agency, for exclusion from families and social networks propelled participants to different belongings, in this case, to the secrecy associated with anorexia. Within anorexia, secrecy and hierarchy create distinction and difference, not only between those who are outside anorexia, but within the ranks of those diagnosed with anorexia. Secrecy, as described in this chapter, does not rely on the polarizations of individual/society that traditional studies have used, but suggests that the dialectics of concealing and revealing are more useful in highlighting the relational and complex transformations that people with anorexia (both individually and collectively) experienced. In people's experiences of anorexia, secrecy (and its power) is an instrumental part of relatedness.

Moreover, my argument extends beyond a disembodied discourse of individual/society, for I was being made aware of a particular sensibility, an ontology of sensations and motives that was often hidden from others. Chapter 5 explores this ontology by analyzing the relationship that participants had with foods. Rather than reproducing well-documented views on the fear of fats and calories as based on avoiding weight gain, I develop a different understanding of the fear of food. Many people with anorexia described foods, and fats and oils in particular, as dirty, disgusting, and contaminating. Others were more concerned to avoid inhaling the smells of food, fearful that the air was carrying calories.

Critiquing and extending both Douglas's structuralist typology and Kristeva's concept of abjection, I argue that it was the amorphous nature of fats and calories, and their ability to seep into and infiltrate the body through the interplay of senses (sight, smell, taste, and touch) that rendered them abject. Fats were the worst food to come into contact with, and a range of measures were practiced to cast out, avoid, and cleanse the dirt and contamination associated with their abject qualities. This chapter also documents how, for some participants, the fear of contamination extended beyond food to other people, fundamentally changing the nature of their everyday social relationships.

Although chapter 5 is concerned with the interconnected relationships between people and food, the ethnographic establishment of abjection forms the foundation of the remainder of this book. As a central theme, abjection pertains not only to foods, but also to gendered experiences (including events, places, and memories). Chapters 6 and 7 explore the ways in which the women in this project experienced their bodies, and bodily processes, as dirty. Menstruation, pregnancy, sex, sexual abuse, and dangers associated with being female (implicitly female sexuality) were all construed as disgusting and too close for comfort.

To feel disgusted, Probyn writes, is "to be fully, indeed physically, conscious of being within the realm of uneasy categories; . . . [disgust] causes the body to hide, to run away from its own cringing self" (2000, 131–132). Disgust motivated participants to protect themselves, clean themselves, and physically disappear. Chapter 7 deals with the gamut of hygiene practices by which participants cleansed their bodies and environments. Bathrooms, kitchens, and bedrooms were the spaces where cleansing occurred but also the places where bodies, food, and waste coalesced, where dirt and cleanliness, pleasure and disgust, came together. It was in these spaces that transformations of relatedness were effected by cleansing (washing of hands, bodies, teeth, and clothes) and by purging through vomiting, taking laxatives, and bloodletting. It was through the passage of fluids (water, vomit, blood, urine, and liquid feces) that bodies were cleansed and, in the process, emotional states of shame, guilt, and disgust were temporarily erased.

Chapter 7 describes the relationships between gender and hygiene, most particularly how gender roles are informed by the persuasive rhetoric and practices of the hygiene habitus. Two points here have ramifications for the entire book. First, the small number of men involved in this project precludes their full treatment as ethnographic subjects. Rather than draw generalized comparisons or conclusions from the limited data on men's bodily experiences,

I include them throughout this book when possible and briefly speculate as to the implications for further research. The discussion of hygiene in chapter 7 therefore focuses solely on the female participants.

Second, the linking of gender roles with anorexia feeds into much of the feminist (and nonfeminist) literature that I have outlined under the heading "discursive approaches." This literature seeks an underlying cause for women being the predominant recipients of the diagnosis of anorexia and assumes that gender relations or certain characteristics of femininity are to blame. While my research takes place in a context that identifies anorexia to be a problem for women, I do not seek to explain why women predominate, or to find the causes of anorexia. My intention is to explore the practices of anorexia in these women's and men's lives.

Seeking to find a single explanation or cause for anorexia is a common pursuit, and in the concluding chapter I reflect on how my research was co-opted by the international and national media into this agenda. Through examples from the print media, I show how the complexities of anorexia that I presented were shaped into simple frameworks. The resultant exoticization and primitivization of my work not only proved to be a grave injustice to the participants of this project, but also highlighted the powerful and pervasive imaginings and stereotypes that surround anorexia.

Writing about Embodiment and Ambiguity

I use the term "embodiment" throughout this book with a specific intention. In criticizing the epistemological pitfalls of Cartesian structures, many post-structuralist and feminist writers use theories of embodiment as a new point of analytic departure. Of these writers, I am indebted to Csordas, who argues that "the body is not an object to be studied in relation to culture, but is to be considered as the subject of culture, or in other words, as the existential ground of culture" (1990, 5; 1994). Rather than take the body as an empirical thing and analytical theme (as the former "anthropology of the body" has done), Csordas argues that a paradigm of embodiment highlights the "existential immediacy" of "being-in-the-world." Clearly drawing from Merleau-Ponty and Bourdieu (both of whom have used embodiment to collapse Cartesian dualities), Csordas invokes the body as an experiencing agent that is intersubjective, relational, dynamic, sentient, and indeterminate in nature.

Stoller warns that early writings on embodiment tend to be profoundly disembodied, and that the sentient aspects of ethnographic fieldwork have been lost through the use of dense and abstract "bloodless" language. To overcome this problem he suggests that "writers tack between the analytical and the sensible, in which embodied form as well as disembodied logic constitute scholarly argument" (1997, xv).[24]

This book follows Stoller's suggestion, bringing to the fore much of what is lost in a textual reading of the body, that is, the smells, tastes, textures, and sensations with which my fieldwork was redolent. At the heart of participants' experiences was the embodied sentience of anorexia: sticky blood dripping from cut forearms, the greasy texture of butter on a tongue, nausea at the sight of food, and hunger as a searing pull on an already empty stomach. These were the ways in which bodies were consumed.

In writing about embodiment one cannot ignore the spatiotemporal dimensions of such a concept. In my fieldwork embodiment was indeterminate in that it was marked by presence and absence, distance and closeness, and things intensely felt and also comfortably numb. Participants told stories that journeyed between intimate memories from childhood, dreams of the future, and the predicaments of their present lives, all of which evoked immediate and sometimes turbulent emotions. Rapport, drawing on Abu-Lughod, suggests that telling stories such as these are "'ethnographies of the particular'—narratives of people contesting, strategizing, feeling pain, making choices, struggling, arguing, contradicting themselves, facing new pressures, failing in their predictions—[that] can be used as instruments of a tactical humanism 'against culture': against that which would incarcerate others in a bounded, homogeneous, coherent, and discrete place and time" (Abu-Lughod 1991, 147–159, cited in Rapport 2000, 89).

People's experiences of anorexia could not be placed into neat, categorical, and homogeneous times or spaces. On the contrary, I was continually struck by the ambiguity of experiences and of the repeated descriptions of exasperated family members and friends who found the disorder confusing and contradictory. Experience, as Wolf notes, "is messy; . . . when human behavior is the data, a tolerance for ambiguity, multiplicity, contradiction, and instability is essential; . . . we must constantly remind ourselves that life is unstable, complex, and disorderly" (1992, 129). The problem, however, is how does one in writing ethnography convey the complexity of experience without losing its very nature? Recognizing this conundrum, Marilyn Strathern writes that "complexity is intrinsic to both the ethnographic and comparative enterprise. Anthropologists are concerned to demonstrate the social and cultural entailments of phenomena, though they must in the demonstration simplify the complexity enough to make it visible. What appears to be the object of description—demonstrating complex linkages between elements—also makes description less easy" (1991, xiii).

Jackson similarly notes that the complexities of ambiguous experience are especially difficult to write about because they are predicated on the simultaneity of double and multiple meanings. Ambiguity, he suggests, challenges many of the conventions of writing ethnography, for it "call[s] into question many of the category distinctions that anthropologists construct for purely instrumental reasons—to systemize their fieldwork experience, identify themselves professionally, and promote the notion that while the world may not be subject to administrative order, it can at least be domesticated and subjugated through logic, theory and academic argot" (1998, 33).

While many anthropologists have written about the semantics and semiotics of ambiguity, few have written of its contingent and fluid nature precisely because it is not amenable to the argot that Jackson recommends (see Battaglia 1997; Jackson 1998; Nuckolls 1996; Throop 2005). An anthropology of ambiguity, Battaglia suggests, "breaks from models that take ambiguation as a textual problem rather than as a *practice* of removing or disturbing those constraints on human relations that categories and boundaries impose" (1997, 508–509, my emphasis). Anorexia, as I understand it, does exactly what Battaglia calls for: it disturbs the taken-for-granted practices and understandings of relatedness. Abjection provides a theoretical framework for understanding these practices, for it allows a theoretical space for ambiguity, for the ways in which tensions are created by the relationships between contradictory elements.

2

Steering a Course between Fields

In the edited volume *Critical Anthropology Now*, Marcus discusses the distinctiveness and juxtaposition of the included essays in ways that parallel the position I have adopted in my fieldwork. The distinctiveness of this volume, Marcus suggests, "lies in the strangeness of the positions in which a number of the writers found themselves in the field. This is not the traditional, exotic strangeness of anthropological fieldwork, of being immersed in other worlds of difference that anthropology itself has prepared one for. It is rather the loss of this condition that provides strangeness here, the strangeness of being immersed in writings, inquiries, and commitments that precede one, surround one, and to which one must define a relationship precisely in order to pursue one's ethnographic endeavours" (1999, 3).

As an object of study, anorexia was a complex and dynamic process that was mobile and multiply situated. It appeared in a network of often-conflicting perspectives: as a physiological state of an individual human body, as a series of embodied experiences, and in representations. As Good (1994) argues, illness is always constituted and embedded in a series of interconnecting spaces, and in this fieldwork anorexia was articulated and practiced through medical institutions, in community health centers, via media representations, and in people's homes and public spaces. Participants thus came to know anorexia through a mixture of personal, social, political, and medical avenues. It was the politics of knowing anorexia—the embodied authority to speak and act—that was at stake.

The first section of this chapter focuses on the complex social spaces in which my fieldwork literally moved. This provides a context, spelling out the initial planning that was as much a part of the ethnography as events in the field. It outlines my conscious strategy of multi-sited fieldwork, which extends conventional modes of ethnography by moving between quite different spatial domains. In these domains I encountered the overlapping and differing sites of treatment, domestic homes and public spaces, as well as the public imagining and representations of anorexia. I not only documented the variety of experiences that participants had, but also interrogated the politics behind the category of anorexia in a number of seemingly disparate global sites. This is the power of multisited ethnography, for it allowed me to move between and across local and global fields and in doing so, explore the "relationships, connections, and indeed cultures of connection, association, and circulation that are completely missed through the use and naming of the object of study in terms of categories 'natural' to subjects' pre-existing discourses about them" (Marcus 1998, 16; see also Hannerz 2003).

The second section of the chapter draws upon Bourdieu's concept of field and related key concepts of habitus and symbolic capital to examine the relationships among them. As an analytical device, this concept is complementary to multisited fieldwork for it seeks to elucidate the underlying and invisible relations in and between social spaces. As Swartz suggests, Bourdieu's field "directs the researcher's attention to a level of analysis capable of revealing the integrating logic of competition between opposing viewpoints. It encourages the researcher to seek out sources of conflict in a given domain, relate that conflict to the broader areas of . . . power, and identify underlying shared assumptions" (1997, 126).

Positioned in opposition to one another, the fields of focus here are those of clinical medicine practiced in institutions, and alternative therapy delivered in smaller community institutions. I examine the various claims of authority to speak about and treat those with anorexia, looking beyond the power of language to examine the embodied effects (and silences) that imbue the category of anorexia with symbolic power.

This chapter thus steers a course between description and analysis, between field sites and fields of struggle. It demonstrates the challenge of constructing an argument through description, and arguing for particular relationships and connections not at all obvious to the seemingly arbitrary category of anorexia. It is concerned with how anorexia nervosa came to "percolate" through a variety of therapeutic environments and the subsequent relationships of positioning, struggles, and strategies that pivot around its clinical reality (Lester 2007, 374).

Ethnography on the Move

To convey a sense of the amorphous nature of the fields in which I moved, I begin with my first sense of doing fieldwork, which occurred during the peak of rush hour early one morning on a crowded bus in Vancouver. I was standing among a group of eight women who were part of an eating-disorder recovery program, accompanying them from the community house where they were living, Lane Cove, to the hospital. As we clung to the overhead handrails, Angela turned to me and said that the journey reminded her of "going to school," backpacks in hand and jackets around our waists in case it rained. After a fifteen-minute ride we maneuvred ourselves off the bus, jaywalked across a busy city road, and entered the side entrance of the redbrick institution, a large, downtown public hospital that ran a range of in- and outpatient programs for people with eating disorders. Once inside, the women became noticeably less chatty and with weary familiarity took the lift to the fourth floor, collected the breakfast trays labeled with their names from the waiting trolley, and sat down to eat around an oblong table in a small dining room.

These women, who came from throughout the Canadian province of British Columbia, were participating in the community residential program, traveling between the hospital and the community residence each day for up to four months. The weekdays of this program were highly structured, with group therapy sessions, body image classes, communal breakfasts and lunches, weekly weigh-ins and skin-fold tests (on what the women called "hell Tuesday"), assertiveness training, and a range of other sessions. These sessions were held on the fourth floor of the hospital, a separate space from that of inpatient acute care, located on the psychiatric ward two floors below.

When members of the group had individual sessions with psychiatrists and psychologists (from which I was excluded), I often explored other parts of the hospital. Sonya asked me to accompany her to the medical day ward on the ninth floor, to help break the monotony while she lay on a bed having her weekly magnesium infusion. During the four-hour treatment, she pointed out landmarks of the skyline through the large window that afforded a magnificent view of the city. Another time she introduced me to her friend Steve, who was waiting for an available bed in the psychiatric ward for the treatment of anorexia. We would sometimes meet to have a cigarette on the roof garden, and when he became frailer and unable to walk, I visited him while he rested on his bed on a medical ward. Steve had agreed to participate in this project but later withdrew due to his declining health.

Twice a week I sat in on medical rounds on the psychiatric ward, listening to the team—dietitians, psychiatrists, ward nurses, occupational therapists, students—outline each patient's progress (or lack thereof).[1] I accompanied the ward doctors on their rounds, visiting people at their bedsides behind closed curtains, observing the delicate negotiations about treatment plans. With permission, I would return later to speak at length with some patients about what it was like to be on the ward, and what this thing called anorexia meant to them. Some of these people were hoping to move on to the residential program once they had reached and maintained their target weight, a prerequisite for living in Lane Cove. At other times I visited the Eating Disorder

Resource Center on the second floor of the hospital, a small, lamplit room overflowing with information for patients, relatives, friends, and the general public. Here I chatted to staff and students who were doing placements, watched videos about prevention of and recovery from eating disorders, and read newsletters, journal articles, books, and pamphlets.

As well as spending time with and interviewing staff from each site, I attended in-service lectures and research meetings. I shared lunches with staff members (secretaries, research assistants, psychiatrists and social workers) at the numerous cafés near the hospital. (Indeed, my first introduction to the eating-disorder team was at a lunchtime picnic on a nearby beach.) I caught buses into the suburbs of Vancouver and met volunteer staff at community eating-disorder organizations and counselors at a family therapy unit. I saw the artwork from an exhibition entitled *House of Mirrors*, an installation of twenty-six full-length mirrors on which the female artists portrayed the impact of the media, diet, fashion, and cosmetic surgery industries on their lives.

At the end of each day, I traveled back to the community house and spent the evening participating in activities or returned to my college accommodation to write up field notes. Although Lane Cove was directed by the hospital, it was not a clinical environment and had the chaos of any busy household. The casually dressed staff took a backseat role, always available in their small office inside the front door, emerging only to facilitate group sessions and eat with the residents. Up to eight people could reside at the house at a time (having signed a contract), participating in the communal cooking, shopping, and day-to-day running of the household. Close friendships were formed, with many residents meeting each other's family members and friends when they were invited to dinner one night a week. For Anna, being at Lane Cove afforded the connections that being part of a family offered: "I really enjoy living here actually. We have a really great group right now—we work together really well. There's no sort of cliques or individuals. . . . I kind of miss it if I go home on the weekend. We have quite a bit of fun 'cause sometimes we go out on picnics or meals and stuff. We watch *Happy Days* in the morning and we make jokes, so it's kind of like a family."

In addition to participating in group activities, I had many formal and informal conversations with the women (including taped open-ended interviews which I later transcribed). In the sprawling, four-story house, there were many corners to which residents took me: down the steep wooden steps to the basement, where the art and computer rooms nestled among the washing machines and boilers; to the wooden table under a large shade tree in the back garden; to sit on beds and floors in the hot upstairs bedrooms and on the porch, where the smokers congregated on old chairs. With anorexia the defining characteristic of the household, the women's seeking privacy for these interviews signaled the private nature of anorexia and its disclosure.

When the treatment program came to an end, a graduation ceremony was held; some women returned to their homes and families, some found apartments to share together, some preferred not to maintain contact for fear of "slipping back into anorexia," and one moved to another country. After completing the program, one woman invited me to her nearby apartment, and on other occasions we met for lunch in a crowded café in the city. Although many vowed to keep in touch via phone, letter, and e-mail, after graduation the intimacy of relationships dispersed. A new group of residents moved in to Lane Cove, and I moved on to a field site in Edinburgh.

Movement was the distinctive tenor of my fieldwork, moving to and from, in and out, and passing through (Clifford 1997, 198). There was no fixed route or trajectory to participants' experiences of anorexia; it was a process in which they felt euphoric, unwell, partly recovered, or increasingly unhealthy.

Where Is the Field?

Abu-Lughod in *Veiled Sentiments* emphasizes the value of researchers' explaining the ways in which they first encounter their field sites. Describing how she entered people's lives in the Bedouin community in which she lived for two years (through reciprocal relationships of guest and daughter), Abu-Lughod reflects on her own perspectives, the type of analysis she sought, and the possibilities and limits of the field. The importance of writing about this initial planning, she believes, is that "the nature and quality of what anthropologists learn is profoundly affected by the unique shape of their fieldwork; this should be spelled out. . . . I do not believe that the encounter between anthropologists and their hosts should be the sole object of enquiry; . . . however to ignore the encounter not only denies the power of such factors as personality, social location in the community, intimacy of contact, and luck (not to mention theoretical orientation and self conscious methodology) to shape fieldwork and its product but also perpetuates the conventional fictions of objectivity and omniscience that mark the ethnographic genre" (1986, 10).

I deliberately chose multiple fieldwork sites for a number of reasons. First, unlike the traditional anthropological field site or community, there is no single geographical location where people with anorexia live or congregate for extended periods of time, other than when they are inpatients. There was no "stable group with which to 'settle in'" (Tsing 1993, 65). In this respect the residential program in Vancouver was unusual, as most treatment programs actively discouraged people with anorexia from spending time together due to the competitive nature of the disorder. Lane Cove offered the only opportunity for me to dwell even briefly in one place with the same group of people.

I chose not to conduct an institutional study, locating myself in an eating-disorders unit, as anthropologists have done in Israel, the United States and

Mexico (see Gooldin 2008; Gremillion 2003; and Lester 2007 for excellent institutional ethnographies). To circumscribe fieldwork to such a site, with access to patients only in a specific time and space, would have limited the understanding I hoped to gain of participants' lives beyond the clinical setting, of their day-to-day experiences of work, study, relationships, and social gatherings. My fieldwork strategy was, as Marcus suggests, perhaps the most obvious and conventional mode of materializing a multisited ethnography (1998, 90).

The notion of mobility in fieldwork has most often been associated with traveling into and out of the field; moving between and across multiple locations is more unusual, Marcus and Fischer suggest: "The realization of multilocale ethnographic texts may entail a novel kind of fieldwork. Rather than being situated in one, or perhaps two, communities for the entire period of research, the fieldworker must be mobile, covering a network of sites that encompass a process which is, in fact, the object of study" (1986, 94).

Certainly this ethnographic mobility is less novel today, as transnational cultural processes (such as migration and the global flows of communication and goods) are central to many anthropological investigations (see also Coleman and Collins 2005; Hannerz 2004; Foley 1990; and Rouse 1991). For me, the transnational process was anorexia—the intimate, everyday experiences of those with such a diagnosis, and the salience and circulation of this medical category in a global context.

In recognizing the fieldwork experience as a process, Clifford (1992) proposes a crosscutting metaphor—fieldwork as travel encounters. This, he argues, is not to reject the traditional concept of dwelling, for fieldwork has always been a mixture of dwelling and traveling (although the rapport, initiation, and familiarity associated with long-term dwelling have tended to remain dominant) (Clifford 1997, 198).

Ethnography, and the fieldwork from which it is evoked, is a dual process of description and interpretation, of examining the connections and disconnections between sites and people and the underpinning cultural categories that give rise to experiences.[2] It is the relationship between sites that brings me to the second important reason for conducting multisited research. Although historically defined by psychiatry, anorexia has had a variety of contentious meanings among the fields in which it is studied. In preparing for fieldwork, I reviewed the competing and overlapping discourses concerning this disorder. The main players came from medicine and feminism, articulating their own causes, explanations, and methods of treatment and prevention.

These differing conceptualizations circulated in all the sites I encountered, to varying degrees, and provided me with shifting lenses through which to view anorexia. Some called the phenomenon I was interested in anorexia, others called it an eating disorder or self-starving, and still others personified it by giving it a name. Anorexia meant different things to different people.

Traveling to, from, and through Field Sites

People with eating disorders can take various treatment paths that, although not mutually exclusive, fall into five main categories: psychiatric wards in public and private institutions, general medical wards, residential community programs such as Lane Cove, counselling and support through volunteer organizations, and outpatient care with community mental health workers, general practitioners, and allied health professionals. Despite the range of services available (predominantly psychiatric), eating disorders are notoriously difficult to treat and recovery rates remain low (Ben-Tovim et al. 2001; Herzog 1988; Herzog et al. 1997; and Steinhausen 2002). Some observe that treatment efficacy has not improved in the last fifty years (Robertson 1992, 70), and that the treatment of anorexia has received remarkably little research attention (Fairburn and Harrison 2003). In light of these observations, I was particularly interested in exploring alternative options to the more conventional approach of inpatient psychiatric treatment.

To select my fieldwork sites, I asked those with years of professional experience in the field of eating disorders their opinions of various international services. I searched through journals such as the *International Journal of Eating Disorders* for program descriptions and sent many introductory letters and e-mails. After much negotiation and information seeking (and several refusals), I distilled my choices to two overseas centers, one in Vancouver and the other in Edinburgh. Both were internationally renowned for their innovative programs, with a range of services from day programs, community-based residential programs, and outpatient consultancies. And both were willing to accommodate me.

What was innovative about both these centers was their focus on outpatient rather than inpatient treatment of eating disorders. This strategy was reflected in the diversity of clinical services on offer in Vancouver, which included ten programs, of which only one was an inpatient stay. I was particularly interested in the residential program, Lane Cove, a specialized service that aimed to provide a safe and supportive living environment for people with eating disorders. The program did not focus on weight gain but challenged residents' beliefs concerning food and noneating and tackled in practical ways the everyday difficulties surrounding food, such as shopping, cooking, and eating in public. The Edinburgh program also treated the majority of clients on an outpatient basis. The staff believed that it was possible to work with people who were significantly underweight, and unlike many programs it did not have criteria for treatment based on weight status. The center did monitor life-threatening situations and respond when needed, but inpatient treatment and weight gain were not seen as a first line of care.

The most innovative aspect of these centers was their dialogue with other fields of expert knowledge, particularly with feminist understandings of eating disorders. Rather than opposing other knowledge or forms of treatment, they readily engaged and embraced narrative therapy, feminist politics, reflexive work, Foucault's theories of discourse and power, and the politics of identity (see also White and Epston 1989). From this backdrop of treatment programs, my focus then narrowed into a closer study of everyday life that involved institutions but moved beyond them into people's homes and lives.

The ease with which I was able to merge these different field sites was telling, for it highlighted the way in which the term "anorexia," despite its various interpretations, was readily understood and transported across international sites. Ethics committees in these locations were familiar with anorexia and granted ethics approval based on the taken-for-granted acknowledgment of the seriousness of such a disorder. Customs and immigration officials did not query my basis for entry to their countries and sometimes offered personal anecdotes about friends or relatives who had anorexia as they stamped my passport. Many participants (including many health professionals) in Adelaide were familiar with the treatment programs I visited overseas and were keen to hear my opinions (and vice versa). Not once during my fieldwork was I asked to explain what anorexia was; more often it was the intersection of anthropology and anorexia that provoked interest. Anorexia was always immersed in a series of constructions and imaginings that preceded and traveled with this research.

Opening Institutional Doors

Despite the variations in the understanding and treatment of anorexia, hospital settings were, in most instances, the initial sites of entry to all fields, as there was no other way to gain access to people being treated in a medical setting.[3] Strict institutional procedures meant that I had to first negotiate in writing, in person, or both with psychiatrists and psychologists (some of whom I never met), community mental health nurses, chief executive officers, program directors, and five ethics committees. In many ways their guidelines and procedures influenced the design of my project.

Selection and negotiation again took place regarding how I would gain introductions to people with anorexia. I chose three sites in Adelaide: a weight-disorder unit in a major public hospital, a program run from a community hospital, and a community volunteer organization.

The first, the Weight Disorder Unit of a major teaching hospital in the southern suburbs of Adelaide offered a number of in- and outpatient services for people with eating disorders. Inpatient treatment took place in a general psychiatric ward, where six of the twenty ward beds were allocated to the Weight Disorder Unit. The three inpatient programs offered were a two-week assessment, a six-week bed program, and a target-weight program. Other services such as emergency admissions and intensive care facilities were also offered. Trained staff provided support and guidance in reestablishing physical health, addressing emotional and social issues surrounding the eating disorder, and reintegration into community life. The unit was directed by a male psychiatrist and included a large team of professionals: rotating psychiatric registrars, a dietitian, ward and community mental health nurses, a social worker, an occupational therapist, a pharmacist, and research staff. I was positioned by the staff as part of the research team.

The second site, at Ashburton Community Hospital in the hills of Adelaide, described itself as a "multi-disciplinary, multi-faceted unit offering more than clinical services alone." This program claimed to be unique to Australia in philosophy and style, and grew out of "the disillusionment of other health workers and consumers with inpatient regimes which exert strict control, restraint and punishment of eating disordered behaviors" (Coopman 1995, 4). It offered an alternative to the more conventional treatment programs run by major hospitals, explicitly subverting the dominance of the medical model in the understanding and treatment of "self-starving" (rather than "anorexia"). The all-female team called themselves "returned soldiers"—those who have recovered from eating disorders. Staff comprised one full-time worker who acted as counselor, physiotherapist, and dietetics manager, and two part-time occupational therapists. The six inpatient beds for those with eating disorders were in the ward with those of women about to give birth, or who had just given birth. Unfortunately, with government funding cuts and amalgamation of obstetric and maternity services, the birthing facility was devolved prior to my fieldwork.

The third site, the Eating Disorder Association (EDA), was a small volunteer-run organization established in 1983 and housed on the first floor of a heritage building in Adelaide's central business district. It provided support groups, a drop-in center, telephone help lines, and education for people with concerns about their body image. It also acted as a resource center for the general public—encouraging people to use its library and view educational videos in a TV room on site, as well as playing an active role in peer and school education programs. EDA also organized eating-disorder prevention programs for the annual International No Diet Day event and Why Weight? Week. Funded by the state government's Mental Health Services (on what was referred to by the volunteer staff as "a shoestring budget"), the service had one fully waged female worker, running on the support of an army of mainly women volunteers. I registered as a volunteer at EDA, working on the editorial committee of their quarterly newsletter and attending some group activities.

There were many advantages to having privileged insight into these centers. I was to be a participant observer (and a volunteer at one), gaining an introduction to the institutions, staff, day-to-day routines, treatment regimes, and understandings of anorexia that each place worked with. I became familiar with ward spaces, the heavy doors that were always closed on psychiatric wards, the smells from the kitchen, and the sound of pool cues hitting balls in game rooms. As entry points, each site gave me access to other social and more intimate spaces of relatedness—people's homes (their kitchens, bathrooms, and bedrooms), informal networks, use of public spaces, and friends, family members, and strangers. Once these relationships were established, the ethnographic focus shifted into what Haraway has termed "web-like interconnections" between locations (1988; cited in Gupta and Ferguson 1997, 39).

The way in which I initially contacted people, which felt somewhat convoluted, was stipulated by ethics committees and individual clinicians. I gave prepared information sheets to health professionals, who in turn handed them on to patients, residents, or clients. If people agreed to participate, their names and telephone numbers were passed on to me by the clinicians, community health workers, or their secretaries. For the group living together at Lane Cove in Vancouver, I made a short audiotape explaining the project, which they listened to at an evening group session. This gave them the opportunity to vote on my admission to the house before meeting me.[4] One woman initially objected (for reasons not divulged to me) but a few days later agreed, and I was invited into the house. At other community support meetings, staff introduced me, and it was often after this general introduction that people approached me and enquired about my project.

The advantage of this intermediary process was that I could rely on established relationships of trust already developed (sometimes over years) between clinicians/therapists and their clients. If people did not wish to be involved, there would be no embarrassment or awkward moment of refusal, as they would not have met me.

There were a number of occasions when gate keeping did not occur; for example, following my presentation to a group of university postgraduates about research methodologies, a young female student approached me to ask if she could participate in my project. Another time a friend of mine mentioned my research in a university tutorial and a fellow student passed on her phone number to give to me, as she wished to be involved. At a major shopping center in Edinburgh, while staffing a health promotion stand for Scottish Mental Health Week, I met two young women with anorexia who had independently come to ask for advice about eating disorders. They started talking to each other, openly comparing notes about their experiences, one lifting up the numerous layers of jumpers she was wearing to prove how cold she was. Naomi was "feeling her way" into treatment, and Jamie had been grappling with recovery for a number of years. Both (who were coincidentally known to the treatment center I was working from) were interested in the project, invited to participate, and included. They left the display together, exchanging phone numbers, anorexia acting as a connecting point for a friendship.

This self-selection process (most often mediated by clinicians) meant that access to people was refracted through an institutional lens. The actual naming of a condition through diagnosis meant that all the forty-seven participants had some level of engagement with a treatment service and had a common diagnosis of anorexia nervosa. By entering the field via a diagnostic system, I immediately waived access to those who did not seek any form of treatment at all (the existence of such a group is assumed though its size and complexion is unknown). Nor did I have access to those who were considered too unwell to be involved in such a project.

Once introductions were made over the telephone or in person, I arranged to meet participants wherever was most convenient or comfortable for them. I drove to people's homes, visited them in hospital, and met them in public parks, cafés, pubs, and shopping malls. Those on hospital bed programs often welcomed my visits as a break in the monotony of being on a bed twenty-four hours a day. Among these was Amanda, with whom I would joke about the numbers she had painted on paper and stuck on the wall of her hospital room, a countdown to the day when she was free to move around the ward. I was always struck by the drama of people standing up for the first time after having been confined to a bed for six weeks—the transition immediately transformed a patient into a person. We could stand, walk, and talk together, leave the room and, at times, the hospital. When Elise was off the bed program, for instance, we drove to the city to go shopping or down the coast to a café. To leave the ward we had to gain written permission from her parents, as Elise at fifteen was considered a minor.

In many respects my project was not dissimilar from Brown's 1991 project *Mama Lola: A Vodou Priestess in Brooklyn*, in which she traveled to the field by car or on the subway from her home in Manhattan. Brown's ethnography was "less a practice of intensive dwelling [the Malinowskian tent in the village] and more a matter of repeated visiting, collaborative work, . . . situated less by a discrete place, a field she enters and inhabits for a time, than by interpersonal relationships—a mixture of observation, dialogue, apprenticeship and friendship" (Clifford 1997, 188–189).

I kept comprehensive field notes in small books that I took with me—a mixture of verbatim quotes, observations (of the setting, how we sat, tones of voices), genealogies, maps of spaces, and my own reactions to encounters. Most often I penciled these "scratch notes" while I was with people. In hospital ward rounds I found it easy to write lengthy notes, as writing case notes and constructing people into patients and was taken for granted in these settings (see also Barrett 1988). When spending time with participants though,

I often pared down my writings to parts of sentences, notes to myself, or abbreviations. My aim was to listen, talk, and engage with people without the constant interruption of writing, which could easily have been misconstrued as the taking of clinical notes and the objectification/surveillance that implied.

As soon as possible after any meeting or event, I added specific details and my interpretations to my notes, keeping my voice on a separate page from those of participants. Sanjek refers to this process as the second stage of field note production—of transforming scratch notes to descriptive field notes (1990, 97). These often exhaustive elaborations would also highlight themes, theoretical ideas, commonalities, and differences between people; follow-up questions; notes on uncomfortable moments (questions or words that raised anger, precipitated tears, or stirred emotions in me); or points in conversations where laughter and joking occurred. I usually wrote these extended notes in transit spaces: in my parked car, on the steps of the hospital, while waiting for a bus, on a bus, in crowded supermarkets or public spaces, and sometimes on airplanes between field sites.

In addition to my field-notes books I had field records in the form of transcribed and printed texts. I transcribed all audio-recorded interviews and conversations along with most other field-note observations and interpretations. These files were then coded (with indexing and a qualitative data program) both for management and cross-referencing of major themes. The end result was a large number of bound volumes of printed field records that included a chronology of interviews, descriptions, observations, my lengthy comments and interpretations, pages of genealogies, documents collected in the field (one participant, for example, had been written up as a case study in a prestigious medical journal), photographs, media clippings, maps of household spaces, written selections from hospital case notes, and copies of personal diaries, poems, and journals. These records, and my field-notes books, became the basis for this book.

My Shifting Identity

As I moved through the field sites, my own position also changed. Doing research in these places meant that I as ethnographer was identified as many things: a guest in someone's home, a visitor in a hospital, a researcher, and a researcher with medical training. I was also at times a friend or a confidante, and on two occasions I became unintentionally involved in suicidal situations that demanded an immediate, appropriate, and ethical response. I was always careful when visiting participants in hospitals, aware that they could construe my casual chatting with doctors and nurses or emerging from the staff-only ward rounds as forging alliances or as discussing confidential information. Confidentiality had different connotations for different people, as Elise explained to me: "I'm able to tell you things that I wouldn't tell them [the staff], as they would write it in the case notes and talk about it at meetings and then everyone would know." Similarly, I was careful not to speak of close friendships with participants to those in psychiatric circles, as the staff had already questioned the wisdom of entering into social relationships with them (which might develop into friendships) in relation to the way in which ethnographic fieldwork was conducted. On two occasions when I was explaining my methodological approach with participants, community psychiatric nurses told me: "But you can't become friends with them."

While the subjects of ethnography are often seen as tactically managing their identity, the positioning of the ethnographer often gets lost or forgotten within the dynamic and contingent circumstances of fieldwork experiences. Like participants, I was also continually crossing, articulating, constructing, and playing down my identity according to circumstances. I was constantly aware of the required renegotiation of my position, a reflexive process that Tsing captures in her descriptions of "walking fieldwork" on the Meratus Mountains of South Kalimantan: "In the process of moving around, I acquired various names, dialects, kinship statuses, and friendships. Certainly this kept me juggling competing definitions of appropriate behavior. At every festival, for example, I had to choose (or waffle) between identifying with the hosts or the guests. If I had friends in both groups who were less than cordial with each other, it was a wrenching choice" (1993, 65).

While I was completing my undergraduate degree in anthropology, I supported myself through work as a registered nurse in the same major public hospital that later became one of my field sites, a situation that confronted me with an especially tricky type of juggling. Although I hadn't worked in the psychiatric ward, I was familiar with the spatial layout of the hospital and the etiquette of ward rounds. Some of the hospital staff remembered me. My subsequent work as a research assistant in a university department of psychiatry as an anthropologist also introduced me to some clinical practices and psychiatric language. Despite these experiences, I was careful not to reproduce the taken-for-granted language and practices that health professionals use, and my positioning as a researcher, guest, and visitor meant that I was treated differently than in my previous role as a nurse. It was through this different positioning that I was able to experience the wards, the people in them, their spaces and routines, smells and sounds, in an entirely new way.

I did not introduce myself to participants as having a background in nursing, as it would have tempered relationships and, I believe, restricted access to certain types of experiences and information. I was interested in aspects of participants' lives that they said they had never been asked about before, and we did things together that they would never do with their nurses. I spent unlimited time with them. I was a young woman of seemingly normal weight,

I had no vested interest in whether they ate or not, and I did not have a set of portable scales in my bag (as some community nurses did).[5] I posed no threat in terms of forcing them to confront or change behaviors. I could be considered one of them, as several suggested. Although clearly I did not have anorexia, it was my positioning away from psychiatry that allowed them to include me in different ways. We often joked about the practices they engaged in, the ways in which they had 'tricked' the staff or perruqued the system—participating in this type of humor was in itself a way of marking me off from others. If my nursing training arose in conversation, I did not deny it, and in fact it was sometimes a point of connection with participants who also had medical backgrounds (five of the women with anorexia had medical training—four were nurses and one was a general practitioner).

Although I considered the relationships I had with many participants to be distinct from my relationships with health professionals, ethical responsibilities were always paramount. On several occasions participants who had given me informed consent to view their hospital case records asked me to divulge what was written about them and their families. While one or two treatment teams were willing to show hospital records to patients (and in one instance encouraged them to write their own comments in the notes), case notes were generally positioned as private hospital documents. Bound by the confidentiality of such institutional systems, I did not pass on any information that I had read in case notes, heard in ward rounds, or discussed informally with health professionals. I similarly did not pass on any information to staff that I had discussed with participants.

There were, however, several occasions when I was concerned about a person's well-being or safety, and I did contact their community health nurse or psychiatrist. One such instance involved Natalia. An evening I spent with Natalia at her suburban home had come to a grinding halt because she had talked at length about a sexual assault perpetrated by her brother and his friend when she was thirteen. It was a shocking attack that forever changed her sense of self-worth and her relationship with food, her body, her family, and all other people. She had waited several months to tell me the story, and this night she felt it was important to speak of it if I was to understand why she wanted to physically disappear, why she was frightened of touching people, of having relationships, and of nurturing a body that she loathed. With each little bit of information she imparted she became physically smaller, tighter, and less able to talk. I stopped asking questions and taking notes and directed my attention to Natalia's obvious distress and suffering. Much later in the night, and after great deliberation and reassurance from Natalia that she would be all right on her own, I decided to leave. Natalia walked me to the front door, and as I stood on the veranda in the cold darkness she slid down the wall in the hallway and slumped on the floor. She refused to close the door, inviting danger and telling me that she sometimes walks alone late at night to put herself at risk. I shut the door and reluctantly left.

The following morning I contacted Natalia's community nurse and explained my concerns for her safety. Not long after this conversation, Natalia called me on my mobile phone to let me know that she had spoken to "her nurse" and had decided to take a few days off work and made an appointment to see her doctor. She reiterated that I should not feel responsible for her emotional response to her "shitty illness," and asked if we could meet again in a week or so. My encounter with Natalia emphasizes not only the importance of and continual prominence of ethics in such a project, but also the potential impact of research on those involved.

I shared as many experiences as I could with participants, including seemingly mundane activities such as grocery shopping, as well as other more idiosyncratic outings such as driving to an antique shop to collect a wooden sewing mannequin that had been put on hold, dropping people off at appointments or the social security office, and going to a theatre performance in which one participant was acting. At the premiere of a short film about eating disorders made by two occupational health students at EDA (in which I, as a researcher, was interviewed), I was surprised to see so many familiar faces. I sat next to an occupational therapist from one of the hospitals and mingled in the foyer afterward with many women (and their families) who had been involved in this fieldwork. It was not that my participants necessarily knew one another, but the commonality of an eating disorder drew them together.

Although the concept of sharing social experiences lies at the heart of anthropological fieldwork and theory, it is not devoid of problems, despite the recent rhetoric of lived experience, or experience-near ethnographies as discussed earlier in the chapter (Desjarlais 1996a, 70–76; Grosz 1994, 95; Hastrup 1995, 79). Experience, like other universalizing epistemologies of self and culture, is based on the principle of unity: "a set of phrasings of depth, interiority, and authenticity, sensibilities of holism and transcendence, and practices of reading and writing have, in the modern era, crafted a mode of being that many in the West call experience" (Desjarlais 1996a, 75).

As such, it is not an existential given but rather a historically and culturally constituted process predicated on continually changing ways of being in the world. Without looking at the ways in which experience is constituted, of its various knowledges, social practices, and multiple possibilities, Desjarlais argues, one assumes an "Esperanto of lived experience," that is, one takes experience "as a fundamental, authentic, and unchanging constant in human life" (1992, 250; 1996a, 72).

Desjarlais makes a clear argument for the reflexive and relational qualities of experience, rather than attributing to it an ontological primacy.

Hastrup similarly emphasizes the dangers of not addressing the reflexive and constructed nature of experience:

> In contrast to a phenomenology of experience that reflects "an experience which, by definition, does not reflect itself" (Bourdieu 1990, 25), anthropology must always question the conditions for experience and explore the "coincidence of the objective structures and the internalized structures which provides the illusion of immediate understanding, characteristic of practical experience of the familiar universe" (ibid., 26). In short, in so far as anthropology takes off in the real social experience of people, it cannot continue to accept radical discontinuity between mind and body, culture and action. (1995, 85)[6]

Experience then, as I use it in this ethnography, is intersubjective and relational; it is not individual and fixed, but irredeemably social and processual (Moore 1994, 3). As Jackson argues: "The task for anthropology is to recover the sense in which experience is situated *within* relationships and *between* persons" (1996, 26, emphasis in original).

Of course, it would be arrogant of me to assume that my position afforded me unrestricted access to people's lives and experiences. There were limitations to what I was included in, and these restrictions were often due to the secrecy and privacy surrounding eating disorders. One young woman became angry with me when I called her at work to arrange a time to meet. In hushed, angry tones she explained that the eating disorder was a very private "thing" and something she did not want her work colleagues to know about. My intrusion into her workspace jeopardized the secrecy surrounding her eating disorder, and she declined to participate in my research. I was always aware that participants shared only what they wanted to with me. While most allowed me to read through their case notes (a request I made only well into relationships), several refused, as they were "too embarrassed" about past behaviors that they knew had been documented in a very particular way. For these people, the possibility of an alternative and supposedly more legitimate rendering of their experiences was a threat to their own authorizations of experience. Revealing knowledge was also dependent on people's health. Some days people were so exhausted that they didn't have the energy to engage with anyone, as I discovered when I went to visit Angelique, who had spent several days in an intensive care unit following a dramatic drop in weight. Another woman explained that she was able to tell me things that she "would never tell a psychologist or doctor because she was 'sort of recovering'" and was leaving behind the secrecy associated with anorexia. She commented that if I had met her several months earlier she would not have been able to discuss these things: "You don't share that until you've left the cult—and then you might be a traitor and tell." Her departure from the collective of anorexia, which I explore in chapter 3, allowed her to explain secret practices. What people shared was always dependent on how close or distant they were in their relationship with anorexia.

Another major area that I did not have access to was people's everyday relationships with family members. While I often met and spent time with family (usually parents, partners, or children of participants), there were limits to the extent of my relationships with them. Only one participant discussed her experiences of anorexia openly with me while her partner was present. More often, I was taken to a private space where doors could be closed (usually a bedroom or living room in family homes), or to the anonymity of public spaces. If parents or partners did come in, it was to ask quick questions (Would we like a cup of tea?), and they often apologized for interrupting. I am not suggesting that participants did not discuss their experiences with family members (many told me they did), but in the context of this research there was an overriding sense that what people shared with me was intensely personal and confidential.

I suspect that the predominance of one-to-one relationships with those with anorexia in this research was due to a number of factors. Many were able to speak about their eating disorders in a therapeutic context (in the safety of support groups or in the private rooms of psychiatrists), and my research was co-opted into this familiar framing of privacy. While we were able to share many events outside this framing, there was a taken-for-granted assumption that what we shared was premised on the intimacy of our personal relationship. When, for example, I met participants in social contexts outside the set fieldwork phase (which I often did), the topic of anorexia often took a backseat or was not mentioned at all. This was particularly the case if other people were present. If the question arose as to how we knew each other, a vague response such as, "Oh, we met at university," would cover any potential breach of confidence. Some participants, however, did not conceal our relationship and openly outlined the context of their involvement in this research.

The other factor that prevented me from observing and participating in family relationships was the associated secrecy and shame, as Carolyn stated: "My parents just blame me for everything. They won't accept any responsibility for me being anorexic. They're ashamed that I've had anorexia because they feel that it's all my fault. 'Look at the others [siblings],' Mum said. 'They didn't become anorexic—it's your fault.'" Carolyn did not discuss anorexia with her mother or sister, and there were many aspects of her experiences that she kept hidden from them. Moreover, like one-third of the participants, Carolyn lived on her own, and it was simply not possible for me to participate in the distanced relationships she had with her family and her small circle of friends.

Ethnography of Diagnosis: Moving Viewpoints

Thus far, I have been focusing on only one aspect of the field, the multiple places in which I conducted research. To leave a discussion of field positioned within a location, context, or milieu is problematic, for it does not reveal the complexities and contestations that occurred in participants' everyday lives.

Fields as Sites of Struggle

Field sites are far more than geographical spaces. They are positioned within what Bourdieu metaphorically terms "fields," the social spaces that encompass a set of objective, historically conditioned relations between agents. Bourdieu defines a field as "a network, or a configuration, of objective relations between positions. These positions are objectively defined, in their existence and in the determinations they impose upon their occupants, agents or institutions, by their present and potential situation . . . in the structure of the distribution of species of power (or capital) whose possession commands access to the specific profits that are at stake in the field, as well as by their objective relation to other positions (domination, subordination, homology, etc.)" (Bourdieu and Wacquant 1992, 97).

A field, therefore, is a structured system of social positions occupied by individuals and institutions. It is also a system of forces that exist between these positions, for it is structured internally in terms of power relations. Positions stand in relationships of domination, subordination, or equivalence to each other by virtue of the access they afford to the capital at stake in the field (Jenkins 1992, 85).

Each field generates its own specific habitus, "a system of lasting, transposable dispositions" that provide individuals with a sense of how to act and respond in the course of their daily lives (Bourdieu 1977, 95; 1991, 12–13). As a theory of action, habitus generates multiple strategies within an agent's trajectory through a field that is not static (Pizanias 2000, 159), and is practical rather than discursive, prereflective rather than conscious, and embodied as well as cognitive (Swartz 1997, 101). The habitus thus functions anonymously and pervasively, "saturating the presence of the world with a field of taken-for-granted meanings which define its practical sense" (Ostrow 1981, 288). Cultural practices, Bourdieu suggests, are produced in and by the encounter between the habitus and its dispositions on the one hand, and the constraints, demands, and opportunities of the social field on the other. The interaction of field and habitus, then, "engages the most fundamental principles of construction and evaluation of the social world," for it creates ways of knowing (Bourdieu 1984, 466).

In the field of anorexia, there were multiple agents and institutions competing for and against the dominant understanding of this phenomenon.

Psychiatrists, health professionals, those given the diagnosis of anorexia, and lay people all vied for authority in this field. These struggles took place not only in institutions and organizations, but in people's homes, in the media, and in the public imagining of anorexia. (I discuss these latter two constructions of anorexia, particularly pervasive and persuasive, in the conclusion to this book.) Everybody, it seemed, had some familiarity with anorexia and had an opinion.

The disparate ways in which anorexia is discursively understood and treated have been comprehensively (and repeatedly) surveyed (see, for example, Bordo 1988; Garrett 1998; Hepworth 1999; Malson 1998). Three main categories come to the fore: historical analyses that argue for and against historical continuity between ascetic practices and contemporary anorexia (see chapter 6); the medical construction of anorexia nervosa; and feminist critiques of the implicit biomedical values of this medical formulation. The arguments between medicine and feminism have created the most contention (see also Lester 1997).

Despite the many variations on the understanding of anorexia within medicine and feminism, the arguments fall into two polarized camps. Malson argues that medicine (in its many guises) "has been largely concerned with producing objective 'facts' about 'anorexia nervosa' as an *individual* pathology; with identifying *individual* characteristics thought to be typical of those diagnosed as anorexic and with seeking to provide individualistic (and often universalistic) causal explanations; . . . [within this context] attention to the physical aspects of 'anorexia'—whether in terms of proposed organic etiology or secondary effects of starvation—has retained an almost exclusive biomedical orientation" (1997, 223, emphasis in original).

Markedly different, feminist analyses are concerned with the relationship between eating disorders and the social construction of gender or with social responses to sexual difference. Feminists' critique of the medical profession's lack of understanding of the gender issues involved in anorexia has led them to set up alternative explanations of the condition. Anorexia (a term often marked as problematic in recent feminist writings by the use of quotation marks) is said to be "expressive of a multiplicity of societal as well as individual concerns and conflicts about femininity, gender power relations, consumption, control and individualistic competitiveness" (Malson 1997, 225; see also Brumberg 1988; Malson and Ussher 1996).

Even within these fields there are contestations, as demonstrated by the critiques of earlier feminist writings (including Chernin 1986; MacLeod 1981; Orbach 1986), denounced for reproducing the medical and psychiatric language of anorexia. These early feminists described what they saw as the oppression of women and the limits of medical discourse and then proceeded to discuss the woman and her symptoms within parameters drawn from that discourse (Hepworth 1999, 63; Robertson 1992, 52). My point in outlining the politics of the field is to explore what Bray terms "an epidemic of significations" surrounding the anorexic body (1996, 413).

What was at issue in this field was the very category of anorexia nervosa; this was the symbolic capital at stake in my fieldwork. Capital for Bourdieu, although borrowed from the language of economics, is not simply the buying and selling of commodities. Rather, it is the logic in which practices are orientated toward "the augmentation of some kind of 'capital' (for example, cultural or economic capital)," which has the effect of increasing status, prestige and authority (Bourdieu 1991, 15). Bourdieu contends that various types of capital can be exchanged for or "converted" to other types of capital. The most powerful conversion to be made, Bourdieu argues, is to symbolic capital—another name for distinction (Bourdieu 1985, 731)—for "it is in this form that the different [types] of capital are perceived and recognized as legitimate" (Harker, Mahar, and Wilkes 1990, 13). Medical students, for example, can convert years of study at a university into the prestige afforded the title of doctor. The symbolic capital attached to the title and the "august array of insignia adorning persons of 'capacity and 'competence,'" such as the white coat and stethoscope, immediately confer a degree of authority and status, as well as the power to diagnose and heal (Bourdieu 1975, 20). The following section explores how the category of anorexia nervosa was invested with symbolic capital and power in various fields.

Fields of Expertise: Fields of Symbolic Power

Bourdieu argues that "all scientific practices are directed towards the acquisition of scientific authority" (1975, 21). Naming a new disease carries enormous potential for symbolic capital in the form of prestige, recognition, and fame: "It is an idle dream of many a physician with academic ambitions to be recorded in the history of medicine as the discoverer of a new syndrome, preferably named after the illustrious scholar so that his name be immortalized" (Vandereycken and van Deth 1994, 153). Indeed, many diseases are named after the doctors and scientists (most often male) who discovered them (Crohn's, Addison's, and Parkinson's disease), much like the early surveyors in Australia who named the land they mapped after themselves (see also Carter 1987).[7] Unlike geographical formations, though, anorexia nervosa did not exist independently of medical language, waiting to be revealed by scientific discourse (Malson 1998, 49). Rather it was constituted and created through the medical discourses that defined and treated it. It was, as Robertson notes, created as an illness category because "it was meaningful to the medical profession—not the starver—a set of symptoms and patterns of behavior which were unreasonable and inexplicable. Anorexia nervosa was rendered an abnormality by a discourse which was privileged to define what was normal" (1992, xiv).

The medical discovery of anorexia is usually attributed to two scientists, the British physician Gull and the French psychiatrist Lasegue, according to Vandereycken and van Deth (1994, 155); each doctor hoped to secure a position as "one of the nineteenth century's Great men of Science" (Hepworth 1999, 31). The question of which man discovered anorexia is entirely irrelevant for my purposes, however. What is important is the language used to describe this discovery process, language that is most redolent of Bourdieu's fields of struggles, competition, authority, and prestige. In their history of self-starvation, Vandereycken and van Deth describe "a race" in which the "competitors"—Gull and Lasegue—struggled to win the prize of diagnostic discovery. It is generally assumed that the "honor" of naming anorexia lies with Gull. It is he "who claimed 'parenthood' of anorexia nervosa" through prestigious clinical addresses (at the British Medical Association in Oxford in 1868) and scientific contributions to prestigious medical and scientific journals (Vandereycken and van Deth 1994, 159). Gull published descriptions of anorexia in the medical journal *The Lancet* in 1888, and it was after this that anorexia nervosa became a distinct disease category.

Once officially named, anorexia nervosa became legitimated, authorized, and instituted by the powerful taxonomies of medicine. As a category it entered the field of psychiatry, and a host of hypotheses and speculations on the causes and meanings of this phenomenon ensued. As Sours notes, the history of anorexia within psychiatry "recapitulates the megalithic history of psychiatry," spanning the four major psychiatric orientations: the biomedical, the psychoanalytic, the behaviorist, and the psychodynamic (Sours 1980, 8; Gremillion 1992, 60).[8] Despite these different approaches, anorexia nervosa was unquestioningly accepted as a psychiatric phenomenon that resulted from individual psychopathology. The influence of this early classification can be seen in the present categorization of anorexia nervosa in the American Psychiatric Association's 1994 *Diagnostic and Statistical Manual of Mental Disorders*, fourth edition (*DSM-IV*). The *DSM-IV* is a guide that sets international standards for classifying mental illnesses, delineating specific criteria that must be met before any given illness can be diagnosed (Gremillion 1992, 69).

The ability to name and classify is for Bourdieu a form of symbolic power. Although Bourdieu did not write specifically about medicine, his writings on religion, law, politics, and intellectuals offer different angles on the same basic phenomenon. Like fields of law or education, medicine is "the form par excellence of the symbolic power of naming and classifying that creates the things named, and particularly groups; it confers upon the realities emerging out of its operations of classification all the permanence, that of things, that a historical institution is capable of granting to historical institutions" (Bourdieu and Wacquant 1992, 167).

It could be argued that the concept of field is another way of describing Foucault's use of discourse and orders of discipline. Yet despite the surface similarities, there are a number of major differences between the discursive production of selves and Bourdieu's notion of field.[9] Foucault's discussion of discourse centers on institutions—prisons, schools, hospitals—and a subsequent theory of domination as self-discipline. Although Bourdieu's field can designate what is often thought of as an institution, "fields are not conceptually equated with institutions. Fields can be inter- or intra-institutional in scope; they can span institutions, which may represent positions within fields" (Bourdieu and Wacquant 1992, 232). Fields, then, are not confined "to particular arenas of agents and activities, such as the family, education, religion, or law" (Swartz 1997, 120–121). On the contrary, they allow us "to incorporate the most mundane details of everyday life into our analyses" what Moi refers to as a "microtheory of social power" (Moi 1991, 1019).

Bourdieu's fields also differ from Foucault's discourses because they are spaces of conflict and competition. This competition cannot be simplified to a technique of domination, for fields, unlike discourses, constitute open spaces of play "whose boundaries are dynamic borders which are the stake of struggles within the field itself." Within this space of play social agents are knowing agents who contribute to resistance, struggle, subversion, and domination, with some even desiring "the condition imposed upon [them]" (Bourdieu and Wacquant 1992, 104, 167). It is thus the movement of fields, their plurality and intersections, that distinguishes them from Foucault's discourse.

Last, in bringing agency and practice to the fore, the interdependent nature of fields and habitus allow gender to enter the discussion. In examining the question of gender as social construction, Bourdieu argues (as many taking a materialist line do) that sex is an arbitrary cultural construction that is used to legitimate and explain sexual difference: sexism "aims to ascribe historically produced social differences to a biological nature functioning like an essence from which every actual act in life will be implacably deduced" ("Domination," 12, cited in Moi 1991, 1030). This arbitrary fact of biology is produced, expressed, and reproduced through the fine-grained details of habitus via embodied movements of gestures, facial expressions, manners, and ways of walking, sitting, and talking. Gender as a manifestation of sexual difference thus appears natural, and the symbolic violence of sexual oppression is misrecognized.

The attraction of theorizing gender in Bourdieuian terms is that it allows writers to reconceptualize gender as a social category in a way that goes beyond essentialist/nonessentialist divides. In taking Bourdieu's approach, "gender is a socially variable entity, that carries different amounts of symbolic capital in different contexts" (Moi 1991, 1036). Gender, like all Bourdieu's categories, is always relational, always determined by its fluctuating relationship to other categories (1038). What Bourdieu offers in terms of gender is a powerful way of understanding both the arbitrary, and therefore contestable, nature of the social, and its compelling presence and effectiveness (Lovell 2000, 15).

To illustrate the relevance of Bourdieu's concept of field and the struggles within and between fields, I describe my introductions to two sites, exploring the symbolic valence of the category anorexia. Gender is implicated in the open play of these social fields and central to the strategizing and struggles that ensued around forms of power.

I start with my initial observations of one psychiatric ward round in a public hospital, for it was this speciality of medicine that claimed eating disorders as "its legitimate province" (Peters 1995, 45). Ward rounds were held every Monday at 11:30 AM sharp in the library, a small room with no windows that was located just outside the entrance doors of the psychiatric ward. Space was limited, and the room often overflowed with students and staff, with several latecomers clustered around the doorway. Attending health professionals included psychiatrists, social workers, community nurses, community workers, dietitians, occupational therapists, psychologists, and a pharmacist—all highly trained in what they call their fields of expertise, in this case, eating disorders.

The first time I came to this meeting I arrived early and sat at the end of the oblong table, perusing the volumes of psychiatry textbooks that lined three of the four walls. A woman arrived (she later introduced herself as the dietitian) and immediately warned me that I was sitting in the chair usually occupied by the head of the Weight Disorder Unit. I moved, and this chair was left free until his arrival.

There was always a distinct ordering to these meetings, with each inpatient presented as a case to the group by the assigned trainee psychiatrist or medical student, although the presenter's eyes were often directed only to the head psychiatrist. This presentation took the form of progress updates for inpatients, or a lengthier reading from the case notes for new patients. In interviews with medical students, Good observes that case presentations offer opportunities for performance, a chance to "be in the limelight . . . gain respect . . . of your colleagues, and especially your superiors." Presentations have a set format, and a "persuasive" and skilful presentation impresses on the audience that the speaker has attained a level of knowledge and "mastery" concerning the patient's condition, the disease process, the diagnostic possibilities, and the appropriate treatments (Good 1994, 79–80).

In psychiatric ward rounds, patients were presented as a biological trajectory, a linear progression from age, weight, stressors, history (including medical history and a developmental history that was divided into social, personal, and family), and mental state examination, culminating with a diagnosis. The language of presentation included medical terminology, acronyms, diagnoses, and medications: OCD (obsessive compulsive disorder), CSA (childhood sexual abuse), ETOH (alcohol) abuse, depression, phobic disorders, amenorrhoea (absence of periods), EE (expressed emotion), BMI (body mass index), CBT (cognitive behavioral therapy), and blood tests involving FBCs (full blood counts), LFTs (liver function tests), and TFTs (thyroid function tests). These presentations could take up to twenty minutes each, with questions and comments reserved for the end, and treatment decisions deferred to the head of the unit.

The vocabulary of clinical medicine, Good argues, "is a highly technical language of the biosciences, grounded in a natural science view of the relation between language, biology and experience" (1994, 8). Although Good notes that language in this context was a performance and "not simply forms of literary representation," he tends to overemphasize it as a basis for power within institutions (81). For example, in describing illness as embedded in social spaces, he continually privileges spoken language and texts. Disease, he argues, is heterologous and is found in the complex relationships between biology, experience, and representations "in the *literature* of the biomedical sciences, in the *conversations* of clinicians and the information produced by their technologies, in the host of '*opinions*' on the condition *articulated* in the social world, and in the *documents* produced by administrative and political bodies which have authority to classify disease and disability" (167, my emphasis).

Barrett similarly privileges language in his ethnography of a psychiatric institution, arguing that patients are constructed through the basic tools of clinical work: writing and talking (1996, 1). Written and spoken accounts of patients are produced through clinical discourse, via the written clinical processes of interviewing and documenting case histories, as well as in the spoken language at case conferences, ward rounds, and the less formal settings such as staff tearooms (17).

This privileging of writing and speaking comes directly from Foucauldian theory, where discourse is reduced to texts and language (Foucault 1972). In institutions, writing and speaking are thus central to the "machines of meticulous observation, examination, measurement and documentation" (Barrett 1996, 17). Douglas similarly contends that the main function of an institution is to name (1987, 101–105). Yet institutions, I argue, have a much broader discursive and active role. Saris, following Lyotard 1984 and Bourdieu 1984 and 1991, defines institutions "as bundles of technologies, narrative styles, modes of discourse, and, as importantly, erasures and silences. Culturally and historically situated subjects produce and reproduce these knowledges, practices, and silences as a condition of being within the orbit of the institution" (1995, 42).

While attention to the literal/metaphorical representation of language is undeniably important (as I have argued earlier), it reveals little of the embodied speaking subject, that is, the "whole dimension of authorized language, its rhetoric, syntax, vocabulary and even pronunciation, which exists purely to underline the authority of its author and the trust he demands" (Bourdieu 1991, 76). Good and Barrett fail to discuss exactly how language represents, produces, and imposes importance and credibility. Manifestations of competence in the sense of the right to speech and power through speech are performances of symbolic power that are underpinned by a host of embodied dispositions.

One of these attributes of symbolic power is what Bourdieu calls "the social conditions of the *institution* of the ministry" that make it possible for someone (and not just anybody) to say, "by the power vested in me." "The real source of the magic of performative utterances," Bourdieu argues, "lies in the mystery of ministry, i.e. the delegation by virtue of which an individual—king, priest or spokesperson—is mandated to speak and act on behalf of a group, thus constituted in him and by him" (1991, 75; see also 1985, 740). A judge, for example, need say no more than "I find you guilty" because there is a set of agents and institutions which guarantees that the sentence will be executed. Similarly, when a psychiatrist tells a patient, "You have anorexia," the symbolic power associated with medicine reinforces the weight of that statement.

Moreover, a person vested with power need not say anything, for it is also by way of silences and erasures that power is wielded. On ward rounds the tacit rules that governed strategies and practices were the measures of competence and legitimacy. In many ways, these rules were unspeakable, for once learnt, they became internalized, taken for granted, and unspoken. The power of speech, Bourdieu writes, lies in a much broader embodied practice than speaking and writing assumes, for it is "in the pronunciation and intonation, everything transcription eradicates, from body language, gestures, demeanor, mimicry and looks, to silences, innuendos, and slips of the tongue that power is performed" (Bourdieu and Accardo 1999, 2).

With this broader view of language and embodied power, I turn to a treatment site in which the power to authoritatively speak about anorexia was legitimated and performed through a different embodied presence.

In contrast to the public hospital's psychiatric ward rounds was my engagement with Monica, the director of an eating-disorder program at a smaller community hospital (the team here had three members). Before I conducted research at this hospital, Monica advised me to meet with the chief executive officer (CEO); our meeting turned out to be a calculation of my positioning within the institution's politicized fields. The CEO told me that this particular program had been "unjustly" criticized and that the hospital management strongly supported Monica's work. In response, I assured the CEO that I was interested in people's experiences of anorexia, rather than in evaluating eating-disorder programs. With this information, and following consultation with the medical advisory committee, my project was supported.

I first met Monica in her office, a large, comfortable ground-floor space that overlooked a well-tended garden. She literally dragged the two large floral couches across the floor so we would be facing each other, suggesting that if I wanted to kick my shoes off and relax, that would be okay. She did exactly this, reclining back on the large couch, explaining that this was what she did with her "clients" to make them feel "more at home."[10] Making people feel comfortable was a high priority for Monica, reflected in the casual clothes she wore and her sense of humor, frequent loud laughter, and casual demeanor. This casualness was best exemplified by a meeting we had in which Monica had just finished a therapy session with a client and was wearing a faux-fur leopard headband that sported little ears.

Monica spoke at length about her own experiences of anorexia and bulimia, legitimating her knowledge of eating disorders through her personal experience. It was a strategy on which she based her treatment, for "if you haven't been there you don't understand it."[11] She characterized anorexia as a journey to the underworld, where the "sufferer" was seduced by the trickery of the male-engendered voice of anorexia. Her descriptions of anorexia along this journey oscillated between the positive characterizations of "a shining angel," "a fiancé," and "a best friend," to the more insidious "enemy," "abusive partner," and "grim reaper." Anorexia was seductive. There were times when Monica would become teary and angry, an emotive display that gave support and credence to her battle with eating disorders.

Monica's characterizations of anorexia as a person or entity with whom she had a relationship contrasted sharply with the clinical language used in the public hospital ward rounds. Her use of language aimed to reauthor anorexia, for it was only through renaming it and personifying it that she could subvert what she saw as the dominance of the psychiatric (and patriarchal) ownership of anorexia. One of the ways in which she reclaimed ownership of her experiences was by using the terms "self-starver" or "troubled eating" interchangeably with "anorexia" (see also Tanzer 1997, 65). These terms were not as fixed as the category anorexia nervosa suggests and included both restricting and purging, rather than one or the other. Anorexia and bulimia, many participants told me, rather than being two discrete entities, were "two sides of the same coin," and many had experienced both.[12]

Despite the differences of authorship, Monica and the psychiatrists both presented their cases for expert knowledge. And each performed that expert knowledge through particular public acts of speaking and gesturing. These contestations represented two extreme positions in the understanding of anorexia. Each field and its occupants were seeking to maintain what they saw as legitimate claims to the understanding and treatment of anorexia. As Bourdieu contends:

> The individuals who participate in these struggles will have differing aims—some will seek to preserve the status quo, others to change it—and differing chances of winning or losing, depending on where they are located in the structured positions. But all individuals, whatever their aims and chances of success, will share in common certain fundamental presuppositions. All participants must believe in the game they are playing, and in the value of what is at stake in the struggles they are waging. The very existence and persistence of the game or field presupposes a total and unconditional "investment," a practical and unquestioning belief, in the game and its stakes. (1991, 14)

Monica and the staff at the hospital both had unquestioning belief in their legitimate claims to treat anorexia. These beliefs were underpinned by claims to specific types of cultural capital (of personal experience and educational qualifications), which could be said to rest on dichotomies such as objective/subjective, male/female, mind/body, and individual/social.

The most pressing struggle in this field was over subjective and objective knowledges, an opposition that Bourdieu sees as "a permanent feature of everyday struggles for distinction and power" (Swartz 1997, 55). Psychiatry is a science that evolved as a specialty arm of medicine during the last years of the eighteenth century (Barrett 1996, 183). Like those of all medical/scientific discourses, its practice is based on rationality, control, and objectivity (see also Desjarlais 1996b). Case presentation of patients in ward rounds characterized this objectivity through the staff's language and demeanor. Anorexia, for example, was discussed in terms of measurements (of body weights and body mass indexes), blood chemistry results, and nutritional intake (caloric consumption). The presentation of people's biographies, which often involved recounting horrific stories of abuse and misfortune, was similarly measured, serious, and "professional" (see also Shullem 1988, cited in Murphy 1997, 4). While I wanted to widen my eyes and shake my head in disbelief at these stories of profound suffering, many staff members remained motionless, their faces not giving away any signs of empathy that they may have felt. The distinctly unemotional atmosphere of these clinical rounds is part of the discourse in which "emotion is constructed . . . as dysfunctional, within the realm of the irrational" (Ariss 1993, 27).

Monica embodied and epitomized the antithesis of this so-called rational mode of knowing. Her personal experiences of eating disorders (including treatment in a psychiatric ward) led her to move away from programs that she considered reinforced male-dominated values of surveillance, control, and power. Her program, she claimed, was vastly different from any others in Australia—she did not distance herself from clients but incorporated them into her life, taking them home for dinner, hugging them, crying with them, and even teaching some to drive a car. Her positioning as both returned soldier and therapist literally crossed the bridge between patient/healer, blurring the hierarchy of power.

Monica was not trained as a psychiatrist and her mode of treatment drew on narrative therapy. Narrative has a long tradition in various disciplinary fields, including psychiatry and anthropology (Hepworth 1999, 113; see also Kleinman 1988; Saris 1995).[13] Narrative therapy, as a derivative of family therapy, gives central weight to the "personal stories" of clients, using language as a site of both individual problems and potential change (Hepworth 1999, 112). In the case of anorexia, clients are encouraged to personify and externalize anorexia, positioning it outside the body. In this process, clients are deemed to have control over anorexia, rather than vice versa. What narrative therapists value are the ways in which clients construct experiences, rather than the interpretation of these experiences as pathology. Experiences of female embodiment, rather than the invocation of authoritarian medical discourse, are deemed to be the most valuable component of this therapeutic skill (see also Robertson 1992, 74).

The professional differences between eliciting and owning stories or narratives was crucial. Monica encouraged clients to construct and manipulate their own personal narratives through artwork and writing, and encouraged them to physically take up more space and speak louder than a whisper. Clinicians who did not follow a narrative therapy style described people's demeanor and body language and elicited, interpreted, and presented interviews as psychiatric case histories. Jackson argues that the spatiotemporal telling of these stories is crucial:

> The most telling difference between the life story and the scientific tract is not epistemological but social. . . . This is because the authority of the scientific essay stems not from a *communis sententia* arrived at through shared experiences of mundane life but from an exclusive knowledge that defines the precinct of a professional and privileged class (Lyotard 1984, 25). Always arcane, always couched in cabbalistic language, always the preserve of an elite, essayist knowledge implicitly divides those in the know from those in the dark; . . . the return to the narrative is a political act (see also Abu-Lughod 1993, 16–19) . . . [for] not only does it imply a critique of metaphysics and transcendence, it attempts to undercut discursive conventions that foster hierarchy and division. (Jackson 1998, 35)

The undercutting of medical discourse was precisely what Monica aimed to achieve.

Another major site of struggle was located in the philosophical values underpinning care. Psychiatry was firmly ensconced in a large medical institution (as a teaching institution it was affiliated with both the hospital and the adjacent university), whereas Monica was located in a much smaller community hospital, removed from the auspices of psychiatry. Monica espoused the philosophies of community health, emphasizing the social, economic, and political contexts of health and illness, rather than locating illness in individual, ungendered bodies. Her clients, rather than patients, were encouraged to participate in their own treatment, for example, by choosing their own meal plans, in an attempt to incorporate them into decisions about their own health and reduce their fear of certain foods. Rather than try and modify people's behavior, Monica would suggest, for example, that if they were going to vomit to do it outside, as the cleaners would be annoyed with the blocked plumbing. For Monica, the treatment of anorexia belonged under the rubric of community or public health, rather than that of psychiatric care.

These vastly different politics of treatment created professional tensions. Sometimes these were conveyed in no uncertain terms, and at other times they were suggested through gesture: the rolling of eyes, loud sighing, or commenting under one's breath or off the record in ward rounds. Some clinicians saw little room for movement between sites, and despite the fact that participants with eating disorders had often tried a variety of treatment options (including both of these), several staff members described "irreconcilable differences" between programs. Staff from each of the opposing treatment sites told me that people with eating disorders would die if they were admitted to the other. The sense of where those with eating disorders belonged was fixed according to specific politics of power and knowledge.

Although these two examples represent the extremes in a range of treatment options, the distance between conventional psychiatric treatment and alternative programs remains vast, both in Australia and internationally. Treatment centers that deviate from inpatient psychiatric treatment are well known to any health professional working in the field. My fieldwork site in Edinburgh, for example, was referred to by an Australian hospital psychiatrist as "that place where starving people walk the streets," or that place "where they let them get down to ridiculously low weights." Hospital programs are equally aware of how they are perceived by others, as one consultant psychiatrist commented: "We are seen as too rigid and too punitive." We should remember though, as Lester (2007) points out in her analysis of an eating-disorder clinic in a small, midwestern city in the United States, that even among therapeutic teams in the same treatment site there may be disagreements as to which approach is going to have the best outcomes.

While this chapter has described two understandings of fields (as descriptive sites and as an analytical concept), it has also demonstrated the usefulness of placing these terms side by side and examining their convergences. As an object of study, the medical category of anorexia carried a set of assumptions that readily translated across continents and allowed me access to treatment sites and people's lives. It was the category of anorexia that connected me with people and places in order to conduct fieldwork. Anorexia thus was already bounded and described before my ethnography began. Yet, anorexia was not a homogenous category. In employing Bourdieu's relational concept of field, this chapter has highlighted the complex and contentious nature of struggles for power and legitimation surrounding the understanding and treatment of anorexia. Anorexia was not a static entity, but one that varied according to people's different positionings within the field. Very different perspectives, for example, could be elicited from psychiatrists in ward rounds and from community health practitioners.[14] Gender, positionings of power, and one's own experiences were all pivotal in how people came to know anorexia. These perspectives were informed by hierarchies of different epistemologies, ways of knowing that were pitted against each other in struggles for power and authority.

The mapping of fields in this chapter, of delineating the relationships between fields as geographical sites and spaces of symbolic struggles, is important to the trajectory of this book. People who were given a diagnosis of anorexia were deeply enmeshed in the politics and powers of these fields. Moreover, they recognized and played with the power of anorexia, transforming this seemingly inert category into a new way of relating to themselves, others, and the world (see chapter 4). Through this research I too became enmeshed in the powers at play, for the relationships that participants had with anorexia and health professionals tailored their interactions with me.

3

Knowing through the Body

This chapter explores my experience with what Rabinow calls the central conundrum of ethnography: how ethnographers negotiate fieldwork relationships among people with whom they do not share a common set of assumptions, experiences, or traditions (1977, 155). These negotiations were complex for me, for they operated simultaneously on a number of levels and were constantly fluctuating. I was not simply observing people with anorexia; I was interacting with them, continually finding common ground and difference, and challenging my own assumptions about food and eating. I was not only entering into new relationships with people, but also entering into a new relationship with my own sense of embodiment.

Here I depict the interwoven nature of fieldwork relationships and experiences. Clear demarcations signal important themes of negotiation: structures of time and space (of where and when I met participants) and the practices of bodily knowledge and experience (how we came to know). This textual strategy is a heuristic device that I use to convey various levels of negotiation, which is a flexible and moving process that continually returns to the spaces between parameters of difference and common ground.

My starting point with participants was on a somewhat tenuous common ground—an interest in bodies and food, and the minutiae of experience that accompanied everyday practices. It was through this convergence that we were able to explore the meanings of anorexia. People with anorexia were often entirely preoccupied with the characteristics and effects of food, with the exact caloric and fat content of every fluid and food. Some meticulously recorded every bodily consumption and expenditure, twenty-four hours a day. They did not take food practices for granted; these were the central focus of their worlds. I, however, came to this fieldwork with an entirely different understanding of food: it posed no threat of contamination, I did not know the caloric value of every item in my pantry, and I could eat almost anything, at any location and time. In Heidegger's terms, foods and all their associated "trimmings" were familiar and "ready-to-hand" to me, mostly overlooked in my day-to-day routines.

Our differences in the "readiness-to-hand" of food practices had direct effects on the establishment and maintenance of fieldwork relationships between participants and me. Participants had very particular routines around food and eating, often eating alone and in private spaces. These spatiotemporal constraints determined the nature of my research, as where and when I met people was continually shaped by their day-to-day routines.

Negotiating relationships was not simply concerned with the pragmatics of time-tabling, however. Although Heidegger did not use his concept of ready-to-hand to focus on embodiment (a task taken up by Merleau-Ponty), by extension it provides a useful framework to explore visceral, embodied experiences of being. As well as participants' different routines around food from mine, I was simultaneously challenged with their embodied and visceral experiences, which were also different from mine. Unlike people with anorexia, I was not aware of bodily sensations, such as food traveling through my body beyond an initial register of taste and smell, or the sheer exhaustion that alerts you to the heaviness of your feet as your legs wearily lift them up each step of a staircase. I had never smelled death on my body as I stepped out of a shower, or felt my parched body to be, as one participant had, "desiccating like a juiceless, bloodless desert . . . [in which I might simply] stop being." Observations and language could convey such experiences only in part, so how could I come to know or glean any sense of what it *felt* like to have anorexia?

The turning point was unplanned and fortuitous: I became pregnant six months into my fieldwork, a state that built analogous bridges of embodiment with many participants. Suddenly my body changed, and my sense of home—of bodily dwelling—began shifting between familiarity and strangeness. My changing body became one focus of interplay between participants and myself and helped to establish intersubjectivity on an entirely different level. Of course, no one can ever replicate another's experience (and replication was not my aim), but my embodied presence in the field was acutely heightened because of my own transformation through pregnancy. It was in this analogous space—in the negotiated, intersubjective realm—that I was able to explore what anorexia, the state of a body in process, could mean for each of us.

Fluctuating Barometers

In her comprehensive book *Food, the Body, and the Self*, Lupton focuses on the development of meanings around food and eating and explores the sites of acculturation that engender eating preferences, practices, and bodily deportment. In this analysis she highlights the commensality that accompanies food practices: "The sharing of food is a vital part of kinship and friendship networks in all societies. The extent to which an individual is invited to share food with another individual is a sign of how close a friend or relative that person is deemed to be. While casual acquaintances may be invited to share a hot or alcoholic drink, perhaps accompanied by snack foods such as biscuits or hors-d'oeuvres, closer friends or relatives share full meals, with the sharing of dinner the highest level of closeness" (1996, 37).[1]

While there is nothing untoward in Lupton's observations and I agree with them, nothing could be further from the experiences of people who have anorexia. The taken-for-granted rules of commensality did not happen for my participants, simply because most people had very different beliefs about the meaning of food and its embodied sensations. During my fieldwork, anything to do with eating and drinking was always negotiated. I could never assume that we would eat together just because I had known someone for a year, or that on our first meeting we could break the ice over a cup of coffee.

Sahlins comes close to the contingent nature of food and relationships in *Stone Age Economics*: "Food dealings are a delicate barometer, a ritual statement as it were, of social relations, and food is thus employed instrumentally as a starting, a sustaining, or a destroying mechanism of sociability" (1972, 215). A barometer is an apt metaphor, as I engaged with people whose lives fluctuated according to what they had or hadn't eaten. Food itself was such a powerful trigger for painful emotions, memories, and sensations that it tailored every aspect of my fieldwork.

Perhaps the most obvious fluctuations of the barometer happened in my meetings with Natalia. During our twelve-month relationship I watched remarkable transformations that were totally dependent on whether she was in an eating phase or not, and whether our conversation turned to food and its associations. Natalia has lived with what she described as "the living nightmare of anorexia" for most of her thirty-two years. We first met when she was an inpatient on a psychiatric ward, where she was being assessed for a treatment program. She was dressed for warmth and comfort in a casual grey tracksuit, a long-sleeved rugby sweater, and white sneakers. Her long brown hair was tied at the nape of her neck, and she wore glasses and no makeup. Natalia seemed hesitant about whether to invite me into the room she shared with three other inpatients and asked a staff member where we should go. The female psychiatric nurse directed us to the quiet of the patient dining room, where we sat opposite each other at the end of a large, white laminated table. Natalia sat in a plastic chair, her legs tucked up against her chest with her chin resting on her knees, her eyes downcast, and her voice barely audible at times. Her body shifted in the chair as she told me I could leave if I found her boring, as she was sure that what she said was really of no value anyway.

Although there was a certain awkwardness to our first meeting, Natalia discussed the more pressing effects of being in a hospital environment, of having to eat three meals every day (and snacks in between) in this communal dining room. For someone who sometimes takes in only fluids for several days, this amount of food made her feel nervous, depressed, and despising of her body. That we were sitting in the only private space on the ward—the patient dining room—although inconsequential to me, had an entirely different significance for Natalia.

After Natalia was discharged from the hospital, she invited me to her home to look at her collection of Japanese memorabilia, which extended to sasanqua camellias and bonsai in her garden. When she was explaining her passion for everything Japanese, she was the most animated I had seen, laughing and excited. But later when we talked about the meal plans that the dietitian had outlined for her to eat at home, she became angry, silent, and physically immobilized. She curled herself up into a small ball on the sheepskin rug that she used as padding for her bony frame on the living room floor, unable to talk and move, sobbing that she hated herself and wanted to simply disappear. Her hands were wrapped around her body under the layers of thick woolly sweaters, her feet curled up to her chest.

The next time we met, I could not hide my amazement at her transformation. She had come straight from work in the city and strode into the busy café in high heels, a short, tight black skirt and jacket, laughing loudly and smiling. Her poise, sweeping hair, lipstick, and jewelry were all in stark contrast to the tracksuits and oversized sweaters she had worn at home or in the hospital. She asked *me* what I'd like to drink, ordered it, paid for both drinks, and chose us seats at the most visible space in the café, on stools at the front window that overlooked the seated patrons and the passers by. Despite much cajoling, Natalia had never been for a coffee with the community nurse she has been seeing for a number of years. I asked her why she was able to meet me publicly, and she said it was because she had decided not to eat and as a consequence she felt "empty, strong, and confident." And unlike the community nurse, I had no vested interest in seeing or expecting Natalia to eat, so it was "safer" and more comfortable for her to meet with me. She drew my attention to the fact that she was having a cappuccino, with "real" milk froth, chocolate dusting, and a sachet of sugar stirred in. This was what she called her "meal for the day."

Illuminating the "Readiness-to-Hand"

My experience with Natalia demonstrated that I could never take meanings of food and its associated practices for granted. The hospital dining room where we first met, for example, did not hold the same resonance for us. For Natalia, it was a place stripped of all potential commensality and invested with dread. It wasn't until Natalia explained what a coffee meant to her that I began to understand the possibility of food having different meanings.

I reflected on the times when I had shared a table with other participants. Ingrid and I always met in the same café in the student quarters of Edinburgh, after she had finished work (she volunteered to work overtime) in a busy retail outlet in the city. I considered the time and space of our regular meetings in a new light. The most convenient time for Ingrid was usually around seven at night. I'd have something to eat, and she'd sip one cappuccino over the next two to three hours. Occasionally she'd eat the marshmallow on the saucer. I came to realize that these drinks were not only her evening meal, but that she wanted to meet at that time as it provided her with an excuse to exit the family home and avoid what she called a "hot, sit-down dinner." I could no longer overlook or ignore a simple cup of coffee, or the different spaces in which we sat, how we moved our bodies, the effects of what we spoke about, or the emotions tied to eating and not eating.

The overlooking or "forgetting" of everyday practices is central to Martin Heidegger's arguments in *Basic Problems of Phenomenology*. In this work he describes how everyday practices are performed without reflection, arguing that they are so familiar that they are ignored and forgotten as meaningful to our sense of being. As he emphasizes, we are so immersed in the taken-for-granted, lived experience of our everydayness that we do not hold it in view: "The world as already unveiled in advance is such that we do not specifically occupy ourselves with it, or apprehend it, but instead it is so self evident, so much a matter of course, that we are completely oblivious to it" (1982, 165).

Part of the reason being-in-the-world has been overlooked, Heidegger argues, is that it is so pervasive; it appears to us only in a conscious way when disruption or breakdown occurs. In Heidegger's terms, as long as the "ready-to-hand" piece of equipment works properly, it is hidden from view and unthematized. He describes such a situation: "When we lift a hammer or drive a car [or take a piece of toast to our mouths] we are before we know it enmeshed in a series of meaningful relationships with things. We take up the hammer in order to drive a nail through the shingle in the roof so the rain won't penetrate; we put on the left turn signal well in advance of a turn so that the driver behind can brake and avoid an accident" (Heidegger 1977, 20).

In short, Heidegger's analysis of ready-to-hand is alerting us to our unreflective mode of existence. For the most part we do not have subject-object relations with the entities in our world. Practical manipulations that focus attention on particular entities and goals force us to presuppose and thus forget the encompassing horizon (Sass 1992, 123; see also Olafson 1987, 162). As a result we miss the meaning that is made intelligible through the linguistic and cultural skills and practices supplied by the world (Leonard 1994, 49). It is only when the taken-for-granted skills and practices of everyday lived experience fail (for example, when one becomes ill) that we become conscious of its readiness-to-hand.[2]

I highlight Heidegger's "ready-to-hand" thinking for two reasons. The first reason is its aptness for exploring the ways in which people with anorexia do not take food or eating for granted. They were all too aware of the "readiness-to-hand" of food—the minute details that accompany every aspect of food—so aware that it dominated their every turn. The women and men with whom I spent time agonized over every detail of food: the thought of eating, when and where to eat, what to eat, how to avoid sharing food, and what to eat first, second, and last on their plate. The process of opening the door of the fridge, taking a packet of cheese out, slicing a piece off, and then deliberating whether to eat it was in itself calculated and momentous. Lara, who was a stage performer, acted out the battle of contemplating putting food into her body through a conversation with herself: "I do challenge my thinking. I go, 'This is a piece of cheese and it's got approximately fifty calories in it. Will I allow myself to eat it or will I not? I shouldn't really because it's fattening, but yes I will because I'm sure I can work off the calories tomorrow. Okay, eat it.' But I go through that with everything."

Many participants kept meticulous records of what they consumed over a day, some detailing the sensory aspects of their bodies at particular times and in particular spaces.[3] Maddy filled her diaries with such intimate and detailed reflexive recordings:

> I love the smells I associate with Christmas. Firstly, the fresh, sharp odor of pine needles—a live Christmas tree is definitely better than those stupid plastic evergreen ones. Then ripe apricots, and cherries, always eaten lots at Christmas.
>
> I have one waiting to be eaten now with my breakfast.
>
> Better still, all these things look and feel (in the case of the fruit) and taste, as good as they smell. What do pine needles taste like? I imagine a sharp small burst of pungent juice, almost of imperceptible size.
>
> There's a correct way to eat oysters, so too there is a correct way to eat apricots. The key with the second is to choose the fruit carefully, and savor every moment.
>
> (1) Enjoy the touch of a perfect apricot, soft, smooth furred skin, more delicate than a peach. The flesh neither sloppy nor hard.
> (2) DO NOT PEEL.
> (3) Smell. Savor the light yet pungent fruity tang for as long as you dare.
> (4) Contemplate the fruit, noting the golden-orange skin, the smooth dividing line. Is the flesh room temperature or cool? Decide the perfect temperature.

(5) This achieved, take a first bite. Do you merely graze the skin to allow the first juices to tingle on your tongue? Or do you sink your teeth straight in?
(6) Eat the fruit worshipfully with the most enjoyment.

The second important reason to bring Heidegger into view is to signal my own concerns about doing fieldwork around a practice that was for me "ready-to-hand." Unlike going to a field site that is immediately unfamiliar, I faced the opposite: understanding the familiar in a very different way.

Eating is intrinsic to my daily routine, and it is precisely the routinization of eating that allows me to be unaware of it.[4] I can plan a dinner for four people or arrange to meet a colleague for lunch, but the memory of what I prepared or the tastes and smells fade in comparison to the importance of, say, why we met or what was said. As Lupton (1996) highlighted earlier, the importance of food and eating was what it allowed me to do. I had come to know it as a way of sharing, as a way of establishing and maintaining relationships, as a vehicle of communication and interaction. The actual mechanics of food and eating were forgotten. I rarely reflected on what I'd eaten, what time I'd eaten, or where I'd eaten, unless it was associated with a special occasion or had some dire consequences. I gave even less thought to how I'd eaten—the sensation of my teeth chewing the food, how my body moved as I brought the food to my mouth, or the satiation of hunger.

Becoming attuned to the presence and details of something that I had for the most part forgotten in my everyday practice was at the forefront of my research. I was already acutely aware of the criticisms of doing anthropology at home regarding the perceived inability on the part of anthropologists to self-consciously reflect upon their own predominant and familiar cultural world.

The critique of doing anthropology at home, however, has a number of limitations that stem from a privileged spatial understanding of the terms "at home" and "in the field." These cultural categories—home and field—denote geographical spaces that are invested with a hierarchical significance. The field (area, domain, or site) was and continues to be the unfamiliar and distant place to which anthropologists traditionally traveled in order to conduct ethnographic work.[5] Home, by comparison, was the place where anthropologists wrote up their fieldwork; it was familiar and close. This spatial separation, which has been subject to considerable critique, is too narrow a concept, for home is not a homogenous space and within concepts of home, the grounds of familiarity and strangeness are constantly shifting (for critiques, see Caputo 2000; Gupta and Ferguson 1992, 1997; Marcus 1999; Messerschmidt 1981; Peirano 1998; and Wafer 1996). The field and home can be experienced as simultaneously strange and familiar, close and distant.[6]

Lucas highlights the spurious separation between home and field in his ethnographic account of people's experiences of schizophrenia in the city in which he lived. Ordinary spaces that he encountered in people's homes, such as living rooms, bedrooms, and hallways, were sometimes rendered completely unfamiliar. They were stripped of their function and transformed into sanctuaries, shrines, and elaborate self-conscious displays of self and identity (1999, 165–166). Walking around the corner from his own house to an informant's apartment was a journey from the familiar spaces and routines of suburban life into a world of interconnecting dreams, images, and realities.

Lucas was not only entering unfamiliar spaces but also engaging with people who had entirely different *perceptions and embodied sensations* from his. The people involved in his fieldwork had experiences that were deemed to be outside "normal reality" (and thus identified as "schizophrenic"); they engaged telepathically with characters on television, had extrasensory perception, spoke to spiritual figures, or were subject to electromagnetic radiation. Some described their brains as being on fire, music vibrating through their bodies, their hearts bleeding, twisted vertebrae, and feeling another's breath within their body. From these extraordinary experiences, one cannot assume that being at home is the same for all, for to do so would be to ignore the range of differences (both spatial and embodied) that coexist within complex cultural settings.

Similarly, the people with anorexia who lived in the city I live in did not share my sense of home. Many did not feel at home in their own bodies, characterizing their bodies as alien, strange, and unfamiliar, yet intimately known. To have anorexia, as Mukai recounts, means having "a different language, a different value system, different ways of interpreting and responding to situations" (1989, 634). This engagement was multiple and in a state of constant flux, as participants and I continually moved between the central fieldwork tropes of distance and closeness, familiarity and strangeness.[7]

Spatiotemporal Aspects of Interaction

The ways participants interpreted and responded to situations often focused on their everyday routines around food. A common assumption surrounding eating disorders is that people with anorexia don't eat. They do, but only very specific things, at specific times, and often in specific places. The diagnostic criteria for anorexia nervosa focus on these specificities. "Food rituals," as they are described in the psychiatric literature (a term taken up with great ease by participants), include "unusual eating habits, for example, food avoidance, playing with food, cutting food into small pieces, using abnormal utensils—a teaspoon to eat cereal, dawdling over meals, making unusual concoctions by mixing food together, increased spice use, increased coffee/tea/fluid consumption, refusal to eat with others or wanting to eat in privacy. Along with the intense preoccupation with food and eating—such as collecting recipes, cookbooks and menus, excessive thinking and conversations about food and food related dreams" (Women's Health Project 1992, 2).

Such unusual eating habits tailored every aspect of my fieldwork. A phone call to arrange a time to meet with someone might take twenty minutes, as it had to be scheduled into a highly structured daytime regime. Tanya described how she planned her days around when she would eat, what she would eat, and the exercise regime in between. She allowed herself to eat only at very specific times, and what she ate—whether it was a few cornflakes or a piece of toast—must take at least an hour to consume. She would then wait an hour before she exercised, which she did for three hours every afternoon, and then wait for an hour afterward. This, she said, was her full-time occupation, as she literally did not have the time to fit work or study into the routine. I asked her what her response was when something unexpected happened to her routine:

> I remember one day Mum wanted me to go out to lunch with her, and I was terrified because I didn't want to go out to lunch and then I said, "What if we have lunch together at home?" And she said okay and that made me feel better, and I'd planned what time that was going to happen and what I was going to eat and all that sort of stuff. . . . Mum was running late and I got so angry. I was almost in tears because I couldn't eat at the time that I'd said to myself I was going to eat. I thought, Why am I so upset about this? but I couldn't stop myself feeling it. Even now I'm sort of rigid in the things I do but nowhere near as I used to be. . . . I just didn't like anything to muck up my routine or my schedule.

One woman joked when arranging a time to meet me, "Let's *not* do the lunch thing," as the trauma of having to eat in public, choose what to eat, and pretend that this was a normal, everyday occurrence was too much for her to contemplate. We always met in the afternoons, and we never met on Sundays, as this was her "eating day." Once she opened a packet of chocolate biscuits at her house, placed them on a plate in front of me, and washed her hands. I (somewhat naively) asked her if she was going to have one, and she shook her head. Although we met regularly and often shared a coffee or a diet Coke, we never ate together over the two and a half years of our relationship.

Negotiating the commensality around food was a constant dilemma for participants. Lara joked about the bluffing that she regularly goes through with friends who do not know she has anorexia. When they phone to invite her to dinner and ask, "Is there anything you don't eat?" she always politely says:

> "Oh, no, no, I eat anything." [Laughs]. And I don't know why I do that—it's like, "I'm fine, I eat anything, but the only thing I don't like is [she pauses] olives." [Laughs]. And I think, Why do you say that, because you

> are no doubt going to be presented with something and you're going to look at it and mumble to yourself, "I can't eat that." . . . I have to talk to myself and [say], It's all right, it's not going to kill you, it's not going to do you any harm, it's a one-off and maybe you won't have so much tomorrow and you won't be eating it again tomorrow—so it's like a treat—just eat it, for God's sake. [Laughs]. And so you do and then you feign enthusiasm and say, "Oh, its lovely," and you get through it as best as possible, but it's not the most enjoyable of experiences sadly, which is a great shame because that's what food is all about—sharing.

My fieldwork was often structured around events and places that did not involve food or the attached social obligations or practical routines around which it revolved. In participants' homes we rarely sat around a kitchen table, and when we did it was a clean sparse surface with no hint of its function. Natalia's dining room was like a museum exhibition, for it was a space of display. On the floor was a Japanese table with four brown velour cushions around it and four place settings, four folded napkins, four sets of unsealed chopsticks, and a circular centerpiece with twelve miniature animals depicting the Japanese calendar years. I asked her if she had friends over to share Japanese cuisine and she immediately laughed at the absurdity of such as a suggestion. The only other table in the house was a round table with a spotless surface belonging to her grandmother, hidden in a corner and waiting to be thrown out. Natalia told me that she didn't need a table to eat from, as she would never use it. She sat on the floor in the living room, walked around the house, or distracted herself while eating as she worked on her home computer. I began to take note of the presence and positioning of dining tables in other participants' homes. Often I found none; if there was one, it was impermanent (a fold-up table or card table) or disguised (covered in papers or clothes).

Another activity participants avoided was grocery shopping. Before I began this fieldwork I assumed that I would be able to accompany people to the supermarket, but for some the thought of going near one produced a look of horror. Natalia refused such a suggestion outright and jokingly pleaded, "Anything but that." She was terrified of shopping, afraid of entering a space brimming with food and indecision and of running into someone she knew. To counter these fears, Natalia would often drive miles to a supermarket in an unfamiliar suburb and carry a small basket that she could abandon if she needed to suddenly flee. The difficulty associated with supermarkets was illustrated in an anecdote that Rita shared with me. In recounting a form of therapy she had many years ago, Rita played with the pleasurable and disgusting connections associated with food and sex: "He explored sex a lot with me [laughs]—intellectually, as a therapist; . . . he even took me to a sex shop once because he thought I must have had a hangup about sex—which I sort of did, but the sex shop was a big yawn. There were gadgets and doodahs in there that I thought were funny. I find supermarkets harder than sex shops."

The trauma shopping meant for Natalia came to light when she offered me a cup of tea and a plate of biscuits in her home one day, many months into our relationship. She relayed how she had bought the biscuits, "whipping in and out" of a nearby petrol station, explaining that the speed of her purchase meant that she could remain anonymous and not have to linger around food. When I left her house that day, she insisted that I take the remaining biscuits, as she was going to throw them in the trash or give them to the neighbor's children. Because Natalia rarely had guests to her home, I became a sounding board, someone to check the cultural rules of commensality with: "What do you do when you have guests? What do you offer them?"

Bettina explained that when she was "at [her] worst," she would spend two or three hours grocery shopping and "only just get a bag of fruit and vegetables." She described why it was such a time-consuming task: "You know the phrase 'You are what you eat?' Well, I took it literally . . . and if I wanted to be perfect then everything had to be perfect that I consumed, put on, did—the washing, everything." I asked how that affected the way she shopped. She sighed. "Oh, dreadfully. It narrowed everything down because the selection process—I'd search through two hundred apples in the supermarket to find the perfect one and think, Yes, this is worthy of going into my body to make me a perfect person. It's horrendous."

The few participants who did shop with me demonstrated the struggles they encountered. It was, as Bettina foretold, a time-consuming exercise in which a variety of very explicit and calculated choices were made. Every packet of food was scrutinized for its fat and calorie content and then compared with the range of different brand names (one woman took her calculator just for this exercise). As well as food, much attention was given to choice of household cleaning, sanitary, and hygiene products. Tamara and I deliberated over such questions as, "Is antibacterial soap better than normal soap?" "Should one have a separate cleaning fluid and sponge for different surfaces and spaces in the home?" My experience of the familiar (and often social) task of going to the supermarket, taking a cart, and selecting items from the shelf with little reflection was far removed from these women's shopping experiences.

Learning the (Body) Language

As Heidegger predicts, it is when taken-for-granted skills and practices fail that we become conscious of an object's readiness-to-hand. When I casually said to a participant around midday, "I'm starving," I got a sideways look and a quick lesson in curbing language that was deemed inappropriate. "You're starving—you have no idea what it is to starve." Similarly, when I was attending a volunteer meeting at the Anorexia and Bulimia Nervosa Association, I was curtly reprimanded for my use of language. We were looking at the program for a conference entitled "The Body Culture," which featured guest speaker Susie Orbach, renowned author of the 1978 book *Fat Is a Feminist Issue*. One of the volunteer counselors asked who she was, and I exclaimed that she was a "biggie," referring to her influence in the academic area of eating disorders rather than her physical weight. I was immediately told off: "We don't use that word around here."

I also learned that a casual greeting could be interpreted quite differently than it was intended. Tanya, who had done a number of weight-gain programs on a psychiatric ward, explained that comments from well-meaning relatives and friends such as "You look great," "You're looking well/better or healthy," could easily be misconstrued to mean "You're looking fat." Moreover, making such a direct link between increased weight and healthiness overlooked the fact that many recipients of such comments could still be grappling with the day-to-day struggles of anorexia. Elise, for example, was terrified to see people when she had reached her target weight, as she found it much harder to explain to people that she still had anorexia. The way around such dilemmas of greeting and recovery, Tanya told me, was to avoid any comments on appearance or connections to weight at all. "Say something like, 'It's good to see you smile' or 'to hear you laugh.' That's better than saying, 'You look so much better,' or 'You look like you've put on weight,' or 'There's more of you.' "

The first time I ate with a group of inpatients on an eating-disorder unit in Vancouver I lifted the lid off the hospital lunch tray and exclaimed with wide eyes that I could never eat that much food. All the young women in the dining room were on a weight-gain program and eating considerably larger amounts of food more frequently in order to attain what was deemed a minimum acceptable weight. There was no response to my comment. Everybody, almost mechanically, went about the onerous task of eating lunch. How to eat in this environment, under the watchful eye of a staff nurse, left me at a loss. Food was not a focus of interaction, of sharing, or of communication. I decided to take the women's interactions as a cue. Yvette sat down one end of the table with her head in a crossword puzzle, moving the book sideways as she slowly lifted the fork to her mouth. The noise of the radio in the small room allowed some to tune out and provided an excuse not to talk. Brianna uncovered each dish on her tray to survey the amount of food and then rearranged the plates so they would fit more neatly. It was a methodical stalling for time.

The conversation was stilted to start with, as a stranger at the table who was researching people's relationship to food was not an everyday occurrence and made all of us, including me, slightly uncomfortable. The young women around the table were as unsure about me as I was about how to eat with and respond to them. Once everyone had finished their meal (which happened within a prescribed time frame), they quickly took their trays back to the kitchen trolley in the hallway and went to the therapy room to lie on the floor for a nap before the long afternoon sessions. I went to the toilet in the same hallway and then remembered that this was not ward protocol, as there are certain behaviors, including going to the toilet straight after a meal, that were viewed with much suspicion by staff and inpatients. In some treatment programs it is explicitly stated that patients are not allowed to visit the toilet after any meal, and that they must instead sit in a television room with others for a set time, usually one hour. This rule was simply to prevent people from purging the contents of their meals straight after eating.

In the community treatment house, Lane Cove, the evening meals were prepared and eaten at the house—a four-story historic home located in the beachside suburbs of Vancouver. The philosophy behind the community house was to reintegrate people into everyday living: teach them how to eat, cook, live, talk, and shop in a communal environment. One night I refused the offer of dessert as we all sat around the large mahogany dining room table. It was a challenge night: ice cream was on the menu—a scary food with which the two women cooking had decided to take a risk. I was repeatedly asked if I wanted the ice cream, not realizing that this was a communal act: to tackle the scariness of ice cream, all had to eat it. My innocent refusal was a rebuttal to the practices of eating that people expected and took for granted in the house. Food in this context was stripped of its meaning as a choice or desire or preference and eaten as a compulsory act. In my refusal, I was exercising a preference that was not available to the others. I had to defend my position later when one of the young women said to me, "I hope you don't have an eating disorder." How I ate, and what I did and said when I ate (or chose not to), was very important to my relationships in the field.[8]

Solitary Practices

The main reason I couldn't share food with participants was that for those with anorexia, eating was a solitary act. They did not eat with their families or friends. They did not like to eat in public. They ate at very specific times and in specific places, often very late at night and in their bedrooms.

Natalia had started to eat in her car on the way to work, a public space but one that had a distinct sense of privacy: "What I've also found now is that I'll take food with me and eat while I'm in the car," she told me. "Like while I'm driving along, then I'll take a quick bite of an apple because I figure that people who are driving concentrate on what they are doing—the road ahead—so they're not going to be watching what I'm doing, and they're not going to be watching whether I'm eating or not because they're going to be concentrating on driving, so actually I find that I do that a lot—a lot more than I was aware of."

The solitary nature of eating was unwittingly reproduced and reinforced by the goals of one treatment program in an eating-disorder unit. While visiting Amanda on a bed program (a six-week treatment program in a single room, where she was required to conserve energy and remain on her bed), I was asked by a staff member to leave the room while Amanda ate her lunch. I hurried after the nurse to ask why they did this, as the only times that I had ever been asked to leave a room in a hospital was when someone needed to do something that was deemed private, such as using a bedpan or having part of their body attended to (an open wound dressing or an invasive bodily procedure). The nurse explained that eating alone was a stipulation of the bed program, for it allowed Amanda to concentrate on the task of eating with no competing distractions. This solitary and concealed nature of eating in many ways highlighted and reproduced practices that were otherwise seen as pathological or deviant.

Participants knew that their food practices were unusual and tried to hide them from others. When Grant was "in an anorexic phase," he would eat only in his bedroom, and in a very particular way. At the house that he shared with his parents and sister, he took me to his bedroom and showed me how he would sit to eat, kneeling on the floor next to his bed and resting his upper body on it. He had taken the advice to "get off your arse, you lazy slob," to its literal extreme, believing that sitting down would make him fat and lazy: "I used to basically walk around a lot. . . . I thought if I sat down I'd put on stacks and stacks and stacks of weight." As a result he never sat to eat and he slept on his side, as he thought that any pressure on his bottom would make it fat. In a similar vein, Natalia always ate standing up in her house because she believed that standing used more calories than sitting. For these participants, you are not only what you eat, but also how you eat.

Every time Grant ate, he would watch the clock in his bedroom, making sure that the food sat in his mouth for exactly one minute. He had been taping a television program about dieting which suggested that you must take at least twenty seconds between mouthfuls of food to give your metabolism a chance to work on each mouthful. The slower you eat your food, Grant thought, the better chance your metabolism has of digesting it. So instead of twenty seconds between mouthfuls, he waited one minute.

Reflecting on these practices (which he no longer does), Grant accepted that others saw them as "quite bizarre behaviors" (as was recorded in his case notes) or, as his family commented, as "stupid" and "weird." Despite protestations from his family (including his sister, who had also been diagnosed with anorexia), Grant continued with what he called "an insane logic. . . . I knew it was stupid at the time and I looked stupid standing up everywhere but I didn't care. It wasn't a problem for me; . . . the whole focus for me was to keep the weight off." To avoid confrontation with his parents, who (somewhat ironically) wanted to "sit down and talk things over" with him, he retreated to the privacy of his bedroom.

Ethnographic Analogy

Community mental health workers knew firsthand the angst that the suggestion of shopping or of eating in public would arouse. Melinda, who had years of experience working in an eating-disorder unit, would often meet with outpatients in cafés in an attempt to ease their fears about choosing, ordering, and eating a meal in a public space. She recounted what she termed an "unsuccessful" lunchtime meeting that she'd recently had with one her "clients" (who was also a participant of this project) that epitomized the rapidly fluctuating barometer of food negotiations. Angela, who had not long ago discharged herself before completing a treatment program, shouted at Melinda when she suggested she try a milkshake instead of the diet drink that she had ordered. The shop owners and customers looked on in surprise as Angela "flew off the handle" in the small café.

Affective Modes of Knowing

Becoming pregnant while doing fieldwork gave my embodied presence an unplanned immediacy. I was at first more concerned than anyone about how my pregnancy and growing physical size would affect relationships with participants, as several had already told me that they could trust me because of my normal size.[9] Some didn't want to touch anyone who was overweight, handle anything they had touched, or even walk in their shadow, as they might be contaminated or transformed. I found, though, that participants made a clear distinction between being pregnant and being overweight. Several were pleased to see that as my pregnancy progressed, I remained "compact, with a tight tummy" and that my tight stomach was "not flabby like fat." Some tentatively and excitedly asked if they could feel my stomach, and others found the swelling and movement too alien. In this range of responses, it was I who became the focus; my body was observed, felt, and surveyed with intense interest.

My pregnancy was a turning point in my fieldwork, for it unwittingly helped to establish relationships between some participants and myself and opened up new directions of exploration. Jackson has suggested the concept of analogy through comparison in answer to his own question, "How can one enter the world of another?"

> Clearly, it cannot be achieved mimetically. Attempting to go native by decking oneself out in the costume of the other can only end in parody. . . . It can, I believe, be accomplished through analogy. Unlike

> imitation, analogy does not eclipse self in an attempt to become other. Its strategy is, by contrast, to have recourse to common images—such as the metaphors of paths and bridges—that are already part of the discursive repertoire of human relationships. Analogy does not, therefore, presume a merging of self and other but a comparison that begins with something already held in common. It is inspired by empathy rather than mimicry. . . . Ethnographic empathy . . . is grounded in engagement. (1998, 97)

Obviously, being pregnant was a totally different experience from having anorexia, but participants were quick to draw analogies about the rapid bodily transformations that both involved.[10] Natalia, for example, said to me one day: "I'm going to say something profound. While I need to put on fourteen kilograms to gain a life, you need to put on fourteen kilograms to make a life." Knowing that Natalia had had several emergency admissions to hospitals with life-threatening cardiac arrhythmias (heart disturbances) induced by lack of food and fluids made her analogy about moving toward death or life indeed profound.

The analogy between pregnancy and anorexia has been made explicitly by Soros, who, having experienced both states, reflects on their similarities and differences: "My stomach had swelled from the starvation, ballooning over my pants to resemble the tight belly of an expectant woman. As my mother tried to feed me, I rejected her, flailing like an infant, pulling my head wordlessly away from the spoon. Here lies madness: the harder I tried to carve history from my body, the more pregnant I became. . . . When I was pregnant, I was revisited by my past. Just as the anorexia performed pregnancy, the pregnancy performed anorexia: for weeks I was so nauseated I could hardly eat, hardly bring in the outside" (1998, 14–15).

For the few participants who had children, my being pregnant opened up discussion about their experiences, of how they dealt with morning sickness, swollen ankles, and feeling fat. Danielle welcomed this commonality and would spend hours reminiscing about her own pregnancy, all the while ensuring that I was warm enough, comfortable, and drinking and eating. For most of her adult life she felt as if she didn't belong, as if she wasn't really "a part of anything." Being pregnant was when she felt "special," she said. "The only time that I have felt that I am like other women was when I was pregnant. . . . I got pregnant and I had my baby and I was the same as everyone else. I did that, and that is the only time that I've felt that I had a place in the world." It was on a connection of pregnancy, of sameness and difference, that Danielle and I based our engagement.[11]

Pregnancy and anorexia were also construed as times when women's bodies become more public than normal, highly visible and the center of attention. Strangers made uninvited comments about both bodily conditions and felt compelled to pass on dietary advice or point out the obviousness of weight loss or gain. Jemma vividly remembers being on holiday in Australia and young men screaming abuse at her from a passing car, telling her she was "a fuckin' anorexic": "No one had ever called me anorexic before straight to my face. It was just like, Whoa! I was really upset and taken aback. . . . I pretty much ignored it. And on the streets here in Vancouver people come up to me and say, 'Do you eat? Why don't you eat?' and I just get stares and glares."

My pregnant body was subject to similar scrutiny from strangers. A man whom I had never met came up behind me at a party and, placing his hands on my bare stomach, said to my friend, "So, who is your fat friend?" People who are underweight or pregnant draw particular attention in ways that people who are equally visible (disabled or overweight) do not.

I asked Natalia why strangers felt they could pass on their concerns about her body size. "Anorexia is close to death," she said. "It scares and intrigues people. We are walking skeletons. . . . Death in our culture is scary, and people see us wanting to die and find that bizarre. . . . They either want to save us or slander us."[12] She spoke of the ways in which pregnant bodies are at the opposite end of the scale, "radiant, in bloom," and about to give life. Both states of personhood are clearly marked by their closeness to something—close to the brink of death and near to term—the beginning and end of life. They both anticipate; they both move toward.

Because of my pregnancy, new interactions and reciprocity opened up to me: explorations of childbirth experiences, sexuality, and giving through food and gifts for the unborn child and myself. Some participants felt the need to feed me, warming cups of hot chocolate to sustain my energy levels or wrapping banana cake in greaseproof paper for later in the day.

Being pregnant was also pivotal because it not only changed my relationships with participants, it changed my relationship and sensations with my own body. Suddenly I had a new identity; I was pregnant and expected to do certain things (give up cigarettes and alcohol). Eating was no longer a mundane, routinized experience. What I ate suddenly became important. I read books telling me what to eat, what to avoid eating, when to eat, and how much to eat. The most remarkable thing, though, was a totally new experience of embodiment. I felt new experiences: I battled waves of nausea when I thought of or smelt certain foods; the sensation of my stomach touching my legs when I bent over was strange; and my sense of smell was so heightened that the air was always heavy with the smells of spring-flowering jasmine, car fumes, and foods. Smell became a primary marker of place and introduced me to new sensations wherever I went. My whole sense of time and space was transformed through this new way of being.

Such changing senses enabled participants and me to play with and explore experiences. When Grace (who is a trained cordon bleu chef) and I spent an hour in a suburban greengrocer's sniffing and praising every sweet and distinct smell of fruit and vegetables, we drew worried looks from the staff. Grace was recovering from anorexia and her sense of smell and taste had returned, and we were both excitedly comparing our heightened senses. Other people also described changing senses. When Rita asked me what it felt like to be pregnant and I described the sharpness of smell, she turned the conversation to her own changed sense of smell since having an eating disorder. The change was difficult to describe, she said, but she likened it to the smell of death—of desiccation—of having no fluids and drying up. She was very conscious of "this sickening and offensive smell," wearing perfume to disguise it and distancing herself from physical contact.

These interexperiences—of the relation between my experience of participants and their experiences of me—were central to my understanding of anorexia. They allowed me to explore not only the observable mechanics of food and eating, but also the important realm of the unobservable—the corporeal and embodied sensations that people with anorexia experienced. This was not to set up two camps, the observer and the observed. Rather, as Jackson (1989) and Stoller (1997) point out, it was to focus on the interactions between us: "Our understanding of others can only proceed from within our own experience, and this experience involves our personalities and histories as much as our field research. Accordingly our task is to find some common ground with others and explore differences from there" (Jackson 1989, 17). Borrowing from William James, Jackson calls this path "radical empiricism," a path that involves activities of intersubjectivity and interexperience—"the ways in which selfhood emerges and is negotiated in a field of interpersonal relations, as a mode of being in the world" (Jackson 1998, 28).

In his ethnography of Songhay sorcery, Stoller similarly argues that even the best studies—such as Evans Pritchard's *Witchcraft, Oracles, and Magic among the Azande* or Claude Lévi-Strauss's *The Sorcerer and His Magic*—are incomplete because they share the same disembodied, objectivist epistemology (1997, 5). They lead us far away, he writes, "from the ideas, feelings and sensibilities co-constituted with the people that these great authors sought to understand." What is often overlooked, Stoller argues, is "the sensuous body—its smells, tastes, textures and sensations" (xv). Stoller's ethnography is far from a disembodied gaze; he literally embodies the notion of "experience-in-the-field."[13] He writes that comprehension of Songhay sorcery demands

> the presence, not the absence, of the ethnographer; . . . the full presence of the ethnographer's body in the field also demands a fuller awareness of the smells, tastes, sounds and textures of life among the

> others. It demands . . . that ethnographers open themselves to others and absorb their worlds. Such is the meaning of embodiment. For ethnographers embodiment is more than the realization that our bodily experience gives rise to metaphorical meaning to our experience; it is rather the realization that, like Songhay sorcerers, we too are consumed by the sensual world, that ethnographic things capture us through our bodies, that profound lessons are learned when sharp pains streak up our legs in the middle of the night. (23)

I was not only entering relationships with people but also questioning my embodied presence in the field. I could no longer ignore the way I shopped, how I selected items from a shelf, the feeling or sound of my stomach rumbling, or the taste of food on my tongue. My fieldwork experiences were thus centered on interactions and interplay with participants, as well as the ways in which my body yielded knowledge that might otherwise have been unavailable (Jackson 1989, 146–149).

4

The Complexities of Being Anorexic

> The body must be seen as a series of processes of becoming, rather than as a fixed state of being.
>
> –Elizabeth Grosz, *Volatile Bodies*

In this chapter I explore the ways in which people with anorexia understood and experienced relatedness in their everyday lives, that is, with how they continually transformed connections by truncating, creating, sustaining, and abandoning them. My understanding of relatedness stems from recent approaches to kinship that have been critical of the traditional divide between biological and social understandings (Carsten 2000b, 2004; Edwards 1993, 2000). "Relatedness," as I use the term, is about the intersection of the social and the biological, which, as Stafford suggests, "refers to literally any kind of relation between persons—including those seemingly 'given' by biology and/or 'produced' via social interactions—and is thus obviously intended to encompass formal and informal relations of kinship and much else besides. The justification for using such a decidedly general term is . . . that the boundaries between various categories of human social relations . . . are often very malleable indeed" (2000, 37–38).

This malleability allows what I consider a fundamental feature of relatedness to come to the fore: its dynamic, divisive, processual, and at times ambiguous nature. The constantly changing nature of relatedness was how people with anorexia understood and explained their experiences, most particularly through their shifting sense of belonging.

The differing and competing knowledges in the field of anorexia brought with them a chain of claims, most notably claims of where people with anorexia belonged—in either psychiatric settings or alternative care. "Belonging" in this frame was premised on what Edwards and Strathern refer to as a "contiguous association of meaning in English, from ownership, to belonging to association to link" (2000, 153). A diagnosis of anorexia nervosa given in a hospital, for example, set in motion a series of placements that designated one as a patient who belonged to psychiatric care and a psychiatric ward; once entered into hospital records, one belonged to what staff termed "the psychiatric community" of people with eating disorders. In various treatment settings (not just psychiatric), people with anorexia were commonly referred to as "my girls" by health practitioners, denoting a taken-for-granted association of ownership, belonging, and gender.

Here I look beyond the discursive naming of anorexia and the ways in which people came to be represented as anorexic to examine the effects of this labeling, in particular how desire and everyday practices of concealing and revealing became central to participants' relatedness. My aim is to show not how classificatory systems of psychiatry were applied, but how participants strategically used them to their own advantage. As one might expect, participants described very different experiences of belonging and identity from those described by the medical or scholarly community. These experiences were not fixed by the identity of anorexia; they were constantly moving and always dependent on participants' changing positions in the field. I am thus concerned with how people with anorexia performed belonging—both through bodily practice and spoken language—toward and away from a psychiatric diagnosis.

Building on established critiques of anthropological concepts of belonging and identity, I argue that there are a number of problems with an inclusive approach to the concept of belonging. Like the concept of home, "belonging" is a term that is replete with sentimentalist overtones, similar to what Edwards and Strathern refer to as the "romantic view of connections as benign and community as harmonious" (2000, 152). It is assumed that the desire to belong to a collective—be it family, community, or place—is a universal motivation. I argue that an exclusive focus on inclusion works to the detriment of exclusion, or rather, the inherent tension of exclusion in belonging. Edwards and Strathern remind us that belonging *includes* exclusion, not in the sense of owning or being disowned, but in operating to cut networks and truncate chains of relations (164).

In the second part of this chapter, I deal with these multiple values of belonging through a discussion of what participants referred to as the "secret world of anorexia." Secrecy operated on a number of levels and extended beyond the simple spatial dichotomies of insider/outsider to the more nuanced processes and performances of concealing and revealing. Secrecy was concealed and revealed in very particular ways. Some participants concealed weight loss practices from all others, reluctant to reveal the intimate relationship that they had with "their friend." For many, anorexia was embodied not as illness, but personified as a friend (and an enemy) that offered support, companionship, and advice. It made them feel "not alone," when they were in fact quite alone.

In treatment settings, however, secrets were often revealed to other inpatients as a way of extending knowledge, creating networks, and hiding practices from staff. These were the social spaces where individual secrecy was transformed into a collective dynamic, through the exchange of secret knowledges and practices, and the formation of allegiances and hierarchies. Although these points of connection had the potential to offer positive support in terms of motivation toward recovery, the revealing of secrets in close-knit therapeutic groups still operated on the basic premises of secrecy—of confidentiality and trust. Anorexia offered new forms of relatedness based on both the concealing and revealing of secrecy, where the associations of sickness were transformed into a productive state of being and belonging.

Outside Anorexia

Estelle was the first to alert me to the complexities of relatedness that were central to experiences of anorexia. The most abiding memory she had of her eight-week recovery program in a large public hospital was one of feeling like an "outside anorexic." I was immediately intrigued by this phrase, as my understanding up to this point was that one either had a diagnosis of anorexia or one did not. How could you, while being treated for anorexia, be an "outside anorexic"?

Estelle explained that she felt like this because she had complied with the treatment program: "I was there eating all my meals and stuff and, like, trying to be really good and the nurses were coming in my room and searching for food because they wouldn't believe me—they thought there was something up." Because of her compliance, she was also challenged by other inpatients with anorexia. "You're not really an anorexic," they taunted. "That," she said, "for some reason offended me because I was, like, 'Well, what the fuck am I then?' If I'm not a real anorexic and not a real, normal person, what am I? Why should I be a real anorexic anyway?" Estelle was simultaneously placed and identified (by psychiatry) and displaced and reidentified (by other patients).

"Outside anorexic" is an evocative term and speaks to the ways in which identity is multiply constituted across different, often intersecting and antagonistic discourses, practices, and positions (Hall 1996, 4; see also Cohen 2000a). Probyn proposes the term "outside belongings" in her book of that title, arguing that it is a theoretical concept created within the much broader theoretical critique of Cartesian metaphysics that I have described. In looking *through* identity, Probyn aims to "speak of something more than the term *identity* can catch." She is interested in the spaces of experience prior to, around, and in between identity, the ways in which people come to belong or not belong, or "how individuals make sense of their lives." Making sense, Probyn argues, "inspires a mode of thinking about how people get along, how various forms of belonging are articulated, how individuals conjugate difference into manners of being, and how desires to become are played out in everyday circumstances" (1996, 5, emphasis in original).

Although in proposing the term "outside belongings" Probyn runs the risk of having her language immediately conflated with the taken-for-granted concepts of outside, hers should not be confused with dichotomous thinking.[1] Her notion of "outside" attempts to "emphasize the ways in which belonging is situated as threshold. . . . It designates a profoundly affective manner of being, always performed with the experience of being within and in between sets of social relations" (1996, 12–13). Thinking about belonging entails, then, thinking about relations of proximity and movement. One wishes to belong or not belong—one moves away from something in order to cease to belong to it. It is a constant process of becoming and unbecoming.

Participants did not say to me, "I am anorexic." Rather their identity was articulated through shifting notions of belonging. Although they were diagnosed as belonging to this specific disorder, anorexia, their sense of belonging was often in between—wanting to have the distinction that anorexia gave them, but not wanting to be anorexic (in fact actively denying that they were). Relatedness for people with anorexia oscillated between these dynamics, and as the following section reflects, was concerned with reconfiguring taken-for-granted ways of relating.

Being Outside: Being Out of Place

Exploring participants' identification with anorexia takes a very different approach from exploring the psychiatric sense of belonging, as they chartered courses that moved from being out of place, to finding a place of identity in anorexia, to fighting to keep it, to moving toward death, to moving away again, and then undertaking the difficult task of trying to reintegrate and belong to a way of life that they had been removed from, often for many years. It was not a simple polarization of belonging or not—they were always mapping out the complexities of belonging, which continually changed and at times appeared contradictory.

For the purposes of "writing belonging," I start with what I term a "biography of belonging"—the narratives participants used to explain how they came to move toward anorexia. "Biography" is an apt term for these narratives, for they were unfoldings of social relations that were constructed from past memories and events in order to explain a presence (see Ingold 1991).[2] People described feeling displaced in childhood, from families, and from origins, and out of place in their own bodies or not belonging to their ascribed gender. In Heidegger's terms they were not "at home."

In talking about belonging, participants would sometimes map out a biography to signal pivotal moments in their lives when anorexia was thought to have begun. Some may argue that the history and origins invoked in these narratives represent precisely what I am trying to avoid—a fixed and unchanging identity located in specific historical moments. But rather than read such a narrative as a return to one's roots, I see it as Gilroy does—a "coming-to-terms with our routes" (1994; cited in Hall 1996, 4). Routes and roots, as Friedman states, "imply travel, physical and psychical displacements in space, . . . the crossing of borders and contact with difference" (1998, 151). This conceptualization of narratives as embodiment of spatial practices or routes (which draws upon de Certeau 1984 and Clifford 1997) is more akin to my general theme of movement and process.

Maria, for example, recounted that she would never sit down and eat her lunch with the other children at primary school—the beginnings, she said, of the development of anorexia. It was often the telling of memories, such as feeding problems as a baby or feeling completely out of place at a family wedding ceremony, that highlighted the ways in which "the processes of belonging [can be] tainted with deep insecurities about the possibility of truly fitting in, of even getting in" (Probyn 1996, 40).

Belonging thus hinges on not belonging, on not fitting in, on being different, on being excluded. Writers including Jacques Derrida (1981), Laclau (1990), and Butler (1993) have already shown that identities are constructed through, not outside, difference. They argue that the "positive" meaning of any term such as "identity" can be constructed only because of its very capacity to exclude, to leave out, to render elements "outside" and abject (Hall 1996, 5). This entails the recognition that an identity is the "byproduct of interrelationships," relational and continually under construction (Jackson 1996, 27).

Exclusion and difference were recurrent themes of participants' narratives. A number talked at length about their feelings of abandonment and alienation from their families, experienced from a very early age. Now forty, Bettina relates that her abiding memory is of a childhood filled with constant exasperation on the part of her mother: " 'How did we ever get you? Where did you come from? You don't look like any of us—you are so different.' " She paints a picture of her childhood as one in which she felt like an outsider: "I was forever told that I didn't belong and that I don't look like any member of the family—I'm totally different, totally, totally different. . . . I knew I was abnormal. I knew that I didn't belong to other groups of people and I used to think that I was alien. I used to think that I was born somewhere out there," and she motions toward the sky.

Bettina knew she was different from other people because she constantly "worried about things." Everything in her environment had "to be perfect"—in line and in order. This included her body, and the only way in which she could become perfect was to eat perfect food and remove every blemish from her body.[3] Her image of perfect was petite, white, clean, smooth, and without defect—like the porcelain faces of the dolls in her collection.

Exclusion and a sense of not belonging to family networks were not always framed in negative terms. In their critique of the concept of belonging, Edwards and Strathern suggest that the positive associations of "belonging"—the desire to belong and to connect—are taken for granted by much of Euro-American academic commentary. Connections, they suggest, appear "intrinsically desirable. People take pleasure in making links of logic or narrative, as people take pleasure in claiming personal links. Linkages may also appear exciting, especially when they cross apparent boundaries" (2000, 153).

People with anorexia confounded such an embracing effect and often took pleasure in being outside taken-for-granted connections. Maddy illustrated this point to me by jumping up off the couch in her living room and returning with a photograph of herself and a group of friends going to a high school formal. She proudly pointed out that she and her partner were visibly different by their unusual choice of clothes, and that many of her friends (including her partner) were gay or bisexual: "See—we are all people who really didn't fit in." The theme of sexuality was particularly significant for Maddy, as over the fieldwork period she confided in me her growing awareness of, and experimentation with, her sexual desires for women.[4]

Others felt so out of place that they believed, and *wanted* to believe, that they were adopted into their families. When I first met Tracey, she talked about the tension she felt as a very young child between her sense of creative identity and that imposed upon her by her family. She remembered having a strong will and an artistic imagination, virtues that were seen as "disobedient" and "wayward" in her strict Lutheran family. Her parents asserted their authority, she said, silenced her opinions, and dampened her artistic flair. As a result she grew to feel alienated from her family and was deeply disappointed to discover that she wasn't adopted. Adoption, she said, would explain her displacement and sense of other identity: "I wanted to be adopted because then I had permission to be different, right. I had permission to feel I didn't belong. I didn't belong."[5]

When I sat with Natalia on her living room floor mapping her genealogy, I colored in the circle identifying her with my black pen. She asked if I was marking her as the black sheep of the family. I explained that I wasn't, but she followed with a long discussion of the symbolism of being the odd one out. "I don't really fit into that family. . . . I used to ask my parents a lot if I was adopted. . . . I can't possibly have been born to these people because I don't match any of this at all. . . . I just asked them all the time [laughs], 'Are you sure I'm not adopted? Because I could handle it if I was—you wouldn't have to be afraid to tell me I was.' "

Natalia, Tracey, Maddy, and Bettina, along with others, were highlighting the fundamental lack of relatedness they felt with their families and friends. Their metaphors of disconnection—adoption, alienation, and sexual difference—all drew on and truncated the powerful and taken-for-granted concepts of biological and social relatedness. Their disassociation was not framed as negative, but as a matter of distinction and positive difference.

For most participants, though, not feeling at home in one's own body was an unwelcome and powerful source of displacement (see chapter 6).[6] All of them with a diagnosis of anorexia had at one time or another encountered their own body as repugnant, some even loathing it to the point of fantasizing about cutting layers of flesh from their limbs.[7] I use the word "encountered" because people often spoke about themselves in the second person. "Your body," they said, "was the enemy, it worked against you," and it was consequently objectified through the language of distance. Although they described a variety of embodied and disembodied experiences, female bodies were overwhelmingly seen as inherently dirty, and as a consequence were, in Douglas's terms, bodies "out of place." Menstrual blood was particularly defiling and polluting, and anorexia played a fundamental role in the erasure and purification of a polluted body (see chapter 6). I was amazed at the number of women who talked of menstrual periods in sheer horror—they winced as they described how they felt when they bled, as if having periods was a cruel joke or torture that they had to endure. Menstrual blood not only signaled the disgust they felt for any sticky and messy fluid, but more importantly signaled an axis of relatedness that operates through women—being desired rather than desiring, danger, the capacity to have children, child rearing, sexual relationships, cooking, nurturing, hygiene. It was this axis of relatedness that did not sit comfortably with many participants.

Being out of place in terms of sexuality was characterized by transformation—either becoming childlike and asexual, or becoming masculine. Several women talked about being "tomboys" and "anti-girl," despising the expectations of friends and family that they enjoy shopping, cooking, or learning how to apply make up. Amanda, who made a point of saying that her parents "hoped she would be a boy," excelled in her employment as an overseer in the male-dominated building industry. This fulfilled her childhood dream to be "more of a boy instead of a girl. . . . I've always been a bit blokey anyway. My friends say, 'You're one of the guys.' "[8] The three men involved in my project were also out of place with stereotypical gender roles—two were gay and the third, Robert, "feared" that he was. Robert said that rather than deal with being gay, he made himself "skinny and ugly" so that he wouldn't be attractive and therefore wouldn't have to deal with his sexuality.[9]

What is central to all these narratives is a profound discomfort with relatedness, with those relationships "seemingly given by biology and/or produced by social interaction" (Stafford 2000, 37). Participants were pointing to experiences and places where relatedness (and its assumptions) was central yet problematic: to families (feeling adopted, alienated), to commensality (sharing food, being nurtured with food as a child), to social rites of passage that connected and transformed people (school formals), to heterosexual and homosexual relationships, and to a sense of relating to their own bodies. These concerns encompassed the wide net that is relatedness and crossed a continuum from the most formal kind of relations (relations of kin) to the least formal (sharing food in a playground). Neither was valued over the other, and at times it was the informal and ordinary ties of relatedness that were highlighted as the most significant. The effect of all these experiences was that participants had the capacity to generate new meanings and experiences of being related, and it is these new forms of relatedness (through desire and secrecy) that I now turn to.

Desiring to Become Anorexic

Diagnosis with an illness or disorder often encourages the diagnosed and their relatives to form support groups and connections they might otherwise not have made. Illness can be a powerful connection of social support. In the so-called HIV/AIDS community there is a strong sense of belonging that is not predicated on a discrete spatial location—it is an identity that has its own powerful sense of connection and relationships through a shared identity. And although that shared identity might be predicated on a medical diagnosis, a bevy of practices and bodily markers also signal belonging to the group. For example, the T-cell count is used by people with HIV to mark significant events in the course of the illness—a low count can indicate decline in immune status, and the opportunity for the appearance of later stages of the disease process such as Kaposi's sarcoma (a purple skin lesion) or pneumocystis carinii pneumonia (PCP). The comparison of T-cell counts among HIV-positive people can be part of the process whereby they "come to a communal understanding of their illness; . . . the count thereby accrue[s] a socially shared set of meanings" (Graham 1997, 61). Similarly, beyond the obvious markers of weight loss in anorexia there are the invisible indicators of metabolic imbalances and cessation of bodily processes (such as menstruation), results and effects that are compared among those diagnosed with anorexia to reveal the seriousness of their disorder.

There is another shared element in this comparison of HIV and anorexia that is not found in other such support networks: a puzzling desire to belong. Several authors have commented on the paradox of "riding bareback" or "bug chasing" in the era of AIDS, that is, the deliberate practice of engaging in unprotected anal intercourse and seeking to become infected or to "gift"—bestow on another—HIV status and identity (Crossley 2002; Gauthier and Forsyth 1999; Tomso 2004; Yep, Lovaas, and Pagonis 2002). People with anorexia similarly talked of the initial seduction by anorexia, and of their ensuing desire to be a better anorexic. There were some who were called "anorexic wannabes"—people who wanted to be anorexic and actively pursued what they called "the coveted title."

This sense of belonging was dependent on context. For instance, being in a ward with a group of other people with anorexia engendered a different sense of belonging from, say, a group of women with eating disorders conversing in a chat room on the Internet (a virtual sense of belonging). Place was of fundamental importance to belonging. If one is exploring the social relations that express attachment between people, one cannot ignore or treat as passive (as Cohen has done) the settings in which these attachments occur (see also Gray 1999, 441–442). Geographers and anthropologists have recently pointed to the importance of "sense of place": of how spaces are created, imagined, remembered, lived in, and invested with meaning (Feld and Basso 1996; Hirsch and O'Hanlon 1995). It is these attachments, struggles, and embodiments of space that interweave to create senses of placement and belonging.

It was when people came together, often in treatment settings or support groups, that the sense of belonging was most evident.[10] At the live-in community treatment setting that comprised part of my fieldwork, the eight young women residents had already had significant contact with a variety of psychiatric services and were well versed in the medical criteria for anorexia as defined in the *DSM-IV* (American Psychiatric Association 1994). This inventory emphasizes physiological and psychological aspects of anorexia, such as reduced body weight, lack of menstruation, and distorted body image. But none of the residents relied on this inventory when describing anorexia (in fact no one did during my fieldwork). Rather they outlined a specific sense of relatedness—of belonging to an identity that encompassed its own particularities of secrecy, allegiance, hierarchy, distinction, language, and practices. These dimensions, as Edwards and Strathern (2000) suggest, go beyond the traditional notions of relatedness as *either* biological or social and examine connections made, in this case, through the shared predicament and desires of those with anorexia.

Within this residential setting some people were trying desperately to belong, to become the best anorexic—to walk into a room, sweep it with their eyes, and know immediately that they were the thinnest in that room. Others were trying desperately not to belong—to recover and leave and have no contact with any person with an eating disorder ever again. Many, though, were caught in a space of outside belonging where they were trying to do both, to be rid of what they described as the "hell of anorexia"—the shame, the guilt and the depression—but unwilling to give up what it afforded them. Staff repeatedly joked about the number of times they had heard this inherent contradiction from patients: "they want to get rid of anorexia but they don't want to put on any weight." The people with anorexia put it another way: "I want to get rid of anorexia, but I don't know who I'd be." They were fearful about leaving the belonging—the identity, the power, the security, and the relationships—that the umbrella of anorexia provided.

The safety that anorexia gave people often meant that it was difficult for them to seek treatment, as this narrative therapist outlines: "Anorexic individuals rarely seek treatment voluntarily. Even if they do show up in our offices of their own accord, they are virtually never asking for assistance in gaining weight, but rather for help in coping with side effects or other issues they do recognize as problematic. . . . Anorexic individuals may deny that they are ill, deny that they are thin, deny that they want to be thin, and deny that they are afraid of gaining weight. They may also refuse to acknowledge that they are distressed, that they are fatigued, or that they are engaging in specific behaviors such as dietary rituals, vomiting, or laxative abuse" (Bemis-Vitousek 1997, 4).

It may have been clear to clinicians (through a person's visible thinness) that a patient had anorexia, but, as many participants told me, they initially denied any sickness, some spending whole sessions in silence, refusing to talk. What participants were playing with, I argue, is agency, a set of actions that shifted according to where they were and whom they were with. Agency, as Desjarlais notes in his ethnography of language and agency in a shelter for "the homeless and mentally ill," "emerges out of a context and a set of practicalities; it is not ontologically prior to them" (1996b, 894). The shelter residents he spent time with "had to act in terms of negation and opportunism. This orientation prompted a form of performative agency characterized by reactivity, indirection, deviation, contradiction, spontaneity and impermanence." This was a political tactic, a strategy "in which people acted in certain ways in order to achieve or gain something" (893).

This strategy, or what Battaglia refers to as "agency play," was happening among participants in my fieldwork (1997, 507). Jackson, whose concept of play is strikingly similar to Bourdieu's notion of strategy and struggle in the field, further explores this notion:

> The existential imperative to exercise choice and control over one's life is grounded in play. If life is conceived as a game, then it slips and slides between a slavish adherence to the rules and a desire to play fast and loose with them. Play enables us to renegotiate the given, experiment with alternatives, imagine how things might be otherwise, and so resolve obliquely and artificially that which cannot be resolved directly in the "real" world. What we call freedom is founded in our ability to gainsay and invent, to countermand in our actions and imagination the situations that appear to circumscribe, rule and define us. (1998, 28–29)

What these three authors are all drawn to are the key concepts of play, agency, strategy, and struggle. It is through these concepts that participants as agents (not actors) continually negotiated their daily lives.

One of the main ways in which participants "renegotiated the given" was through a reformulation of desire. Because anorexia was viewed as a desirable positioning by many of the people who had the diagnosis and was a goal they often strove toward, a number who knew that they were being admitted to a psychiatric unit for assessment tried desperately to lose as much weight as they could before admission so they wouldn't be laughed at as a fraud or a joke. One woman told the staff that she couldn't be admitted for three weeks because of work commitments, while admitting to me that she really wanted the time to reduce her weight to thirty-five kilograms (seventy-seven pounds) and so be justifiably treated as "an anorexic." The distinction accompanying authentic diagnosis (and not a failed anorexic) was paramount. Another who usually planned to lose weight before going to the hospital explained that this practice was "a bit like cleaning your house before the cleaner comes." People wanted to clearly show by their bodies that they deserved to be called anorexic.

The desire to be the best anorexic was exemplified by Amanda, a thirty-year-old woman who had lived with anorexia, depression, and self-abuse since her teenage years. Despite multiple admissions to private and public hospitals over the last sixteen years, Amanda told me of her continuing desire to be a "better anorexic." From her hospital bed—where she was supposedly recovering—she compared herself with two of the most widely publicized women with anorexia, the identical twins Samantha and Michaela Kendall from Birmingham, England, whose battle with anorexia was highly publicized in the media throughout the nineties:

> I wanted to be noticed. I wanted to be different. And I still want to be different, and that's one of the reasons I don't want to put on the weight because I don't want to look normal, I don't want to look like everyone else. . . . You're always trying to be the best anorexic, so you always try to outcompete anyone that you know and meet. I guess you read about those twins in England and you think, Wow, they were really good at this; I wish I could be as good as them. I wanted to be as strong as them and as good as them; . . . they looked disgusting but it was, like, Why do I even think I'm sick? It's a joke to think I'm sick because I'm just so much healthier than everyone else. Look at them—they're so thin. And it's like I'm just not even sick because I'm not as thin as them, and until I can be thinner or sicker than other people I can't prove it to myself. I still don't think that I've been sick enough and that's the problem.

Graphic pictures of the Kendall twins appeared regularly in popular Australian women's magazines throughout the nineties, and interviews were recorded when the women were at extremely low weights on daytime U.S. chat shows such as *The Oprah Winfrey Show*. Michaela died in 1994 and Samantha the following year.

To be seriously ill was not a deterrent for participants. On the contrary, serious medical conditions related to complications of low weight simply gave more credibility to the distinction of anorexia, to playing on that fine line between life and death. To gain access to anorexia, Sonya recounted, "you have to be really thin and you have to be really sick—the sickest they've ever seen. . . . See, if you're ninety pounds, that's not good enough to be in the cult." To have a heart attack due to low levels of potassium, for example, was a legitimate entry card.

Participants said that the hardest question for others to deal with was why *young* people (mainly women) would desire to literally starve themselves to death. "Just eat! What's wrong with you, just eat!" implored families and friends. Desiring death is the ultimate negation of relatedness and was seen as a lack of reason, for in desiring anorexia and moving toward death participants were confounding an underpinning philosophy that privileged rationality and progress. Western medicine, as Foucault and others have argued, is founded on the bedrock of rationality and progress, by which bodies and diseases are categorized, ordered, and treated (with the aim to assist or cure). The flouting of this philosophy may be partly responsible for the negative attitudes toward people with eating disorders by some health professionals. In their study concerning professional attitudes to people with eating disorders, Cameron, Willi, and Richter reported a high level of frustration, fear, anxiety, and helplessness: "It's like beating your head against a brick wall; . . . they [the patients] are not prepared to follow the path you are laying open for them [and] . . . nothing seems to get through to them" (1997, 28).

The two participants in my research who perhaps most graphically played out this scenario were Danielle and Charlotte, both of whom struggled with their desire to have anorexia despite repeated warnings that they could irreparably damage their health. Both had insulin-dependent diabetes and skipped doses of insulin in order to rapidly lose weight. They told me that the desire to be empty and pure outweighed the complications of diabetes (risks such as reduced blood circulation to the peripheral parts of the body). During the course of my research both women lost their eyesight as a result of these actions, a loss made even more poignant by Charlotte's being a visual artist and Danielle the single mother of a young child.[11]

The ways in which desire moves the bodies of some people diagnosed with anorexia is antithetical to the Western philosophical tradition that has, as Nietzsche points out, tended to fear "appearance, change, pain, death, the corporeal, the senses, fate and bondage, the aimless." And this, for Nietzsche, is the underlying problem: "We remain entangled in error, necessitated to error, to precisely the extent that our prejudice in favor of reason compels us to posit unity, identity, duration, substance, cause, materiality and being" in a search for the immutable (1968, 220, cited in Dollimore 1998, 245).

Desiring anorexia was not entirely a negative process for participants. Rather than being a lack or an absent negative (as Kristeva and psychoanalysis more generally has positioned it), desire was also experienced as a series of practices that produced, connected, separated, and constituted social relations (Grosz 1994, 165).[12] Desire was an important dimension of participants' social lives, for, as Probyn argues, "it is through and with desire that we figure relations of proximity to others and other forms of sociality. It is what remakes the social as a dynamic proposition, for if we live within a grid or network of different points, we live through desire to make them connect differently" (1996, 13).

One of the most recent illustrations of the building of social relations through the desire to have or be a better anorexic is evidenced by the ever-increasing number of pro-anorexic Web sites. These Web sites (among them, *The Purgatorium*, *Starving for Perfection*, *Wasting Away on the Web*, *Dying to Be Thin*, *Anorexic with Pride*, and *Goddess Ana*) are constructed by people with anorexia and offer advice such as "how to improve your eating disorder, and how to deceive your family and friends." Beautiful by Bones describes itself as a club for sharing tips, being pro-anorexic, and "being beautiful by having your bones show loud and proud." Photographs of emaciated women (such as Karen Carpenter) and men are posted as "thinspiration," as desired states of being. E-mail groups also promote anorexia; Puking Pals, for example, sums up its philosophy as "how to have your cake and puke it."

While there has been public outrage about the ethical and moral responsibilities of these Web site authors and their Internet site providers (in the past Yahoo has agreed to remove some such sites), these Web sites demonstrate a very particular playing with agency. Cyberspace offers a space to simultaneously reveal and conceal information. People with anorexia were able to project incredibly intimate and mundane aspects of their daily lives into such a public arena precisely because of the anonymity it provided (Dias 2003; Fox, Ward, and O'Rourke 2005). They described experiences and practices that, in a different context, would be pathologized, admonished, or censured. This was a strategic use of technology in which agency was strategically revealed yet concealed.

It was this playing with agency that ignited public outrage. It was, for example, no longer medical practitioners or health professionals who were the experts, but the people with anorexia themselves, as this warning from the anonymous "eating disordered" "Sammy" details:

> If you are using Syrup of Ipecac or Laxatives as a means of weight loss, or are considering using either of these methods, then you NEED to read this page.
>
> Syrup of Ipecac is meant for EMERGENCY ROOMS or HOUSEHOLD EMERGENCIES ONLY! Its purpose is to save the life of someone who has ingested poison, and induces vomiting to rid the victim of the poison. This is its purpose, and should be its only purpose. I know some of you are curious about Ipecac, are considering using it as a means of purging, or are actually using it at present. What I would say to you, is DONT. For your own sake, DONT. I have been through years of bulimia. I know how desperate you get, just to rid yourself of the food which is "raping" you and contaminating ur [sic] stomach. Ipecac is not the answer. If you must, use your fingers or a toothbrush, etc.

This playing, Battaglia argues, "is useful to people not so much for controlling or determining a site of authorship or authority as for ambiguating authorship or authority." As a form of play, agency is thus "a vehicle or site for problematizing sociality" (1997, 506). The authors of these Web sites knew that they were problematizing sociality and warned visitors that the information would be of interest only to those who desired to be anorexic or to maintain anorexia, not to family members, friends, or those recovering from eating disorders. These sites graphically illustrate the ways in which people with anorexia renegotiate the taken-for-granted nature of illness, agency, desire, and relatedness.

Creating Relatedness through Concealing and Revealing

Estelle experienced the reconfiguration of desire, power, and belonging through her exposure to the social relations of secrecy in eating disorders. She was amazed when she was first admitted to an inpatient program and met with other anorexic patients: "I found that there was a whole culture behind anorexia, once I got in there. There was this whole culture thing. They all seem to stick together and they have their laxative abuse and stuff like that, but it's almost like a trade secret—like it was really bizarre for me. Because I'd never really known anyone with eating disorders while I'd had it, but I knew about this whole thing because I'd been warned about getting sucked into the whole anorexia culture and the girls that didn't want to get better."

Estelle's experience at the hospital highlights the tensions of allegiance, of wanting to recover and conform to her program and of being maligned by other patients for doing so: "I wanted to fit into that culture when I went to the hospital because I wanted to fit in with everyone, and they all saw me as this freak that wants to get better and at first I felt really rejected by them. . . . I was leaving the thing [anorexia], so they didn't like me that much." Even though Estelle's nonconformity puzzled the group, they took great delight in introducing her to the collective ways of anorexia. When they discovered she hadn't used laxatives to lose weight, they explained the practice to her, tempering their information with a plea for anonymity—"We haven't really told you about this, okay?"

I had already gleaned from health professionals that there was an element of concealment surrounding anorexia. During ward rounds at one major hospital, the dietitian would report on each patient's weight status. It was not unusual for some patients who were on weight-gain programs to register an initial weight loss due to fluid loss. Continued weight loss, however, was viewed with much suspicion. There were cries of cheating and lying, and it was immediately assumed that the patients must be hiding food and secretly exercising. Measures were put in place to counteract cheating. A total of three warnings was given to patients who were contravening their contracts, with the common offending behaviors being hiding or secretly disposing of food or surreptitiously exercising. Rooms and belongings could be searched to find hidden items, such as laxatives or unwanted food.

Outside treatment settings, those in my project were reluctant to reveal practices of weight loss or food refusal to those around them. Family and friends were often not aware of the extent to which a participant had gone to reduce her weight. Rita recalled the strain of having to live "like a criminal—you have to constantly hide and lie and cheat." She explained that being anorexic "was like having a full-time job . . . because there's deception involved. Not only do you have to make your environment exactly how it should be and control what you put in your mouth, but you also have to deceive other people and especially now they know what I do. . . . In the early days, certainly in my twenties when I went to parties or dinners, I used to feel enormously proud if I could get through the evening without eating anything, if I was driving home or going home and I could say to myself, Phew, I got out of eating and no one noticed." When I asked her how she could do that, she replied:

> Oh, there are lots of ways. You pretend to eat, for a start. You put your fork in something—you hold it like this (holds the fork in her hand near her face), then it goes on around you, and then you put it down again. You blend in—it's like part of a movie. But nothing's changing on your plate—you're moving food around, but it's still there. You can make it look as though you've made a dent—and you do it as inconspicuously as you can—and then you take your plate back into the kitchen and scrape it into the bin. It's a strain because you constantly have to be assessing and playing the room like some bloody entertainer so as not to be—sort

> of like the reverse, because you don't want to be noticed and so you play the room in such a way as not to be noticed that you're cheating. It's a lie, it's a cheat, it's a hustle—it's a strain. But then at the end of it, if you succeed, you feel good.

These tactics of concealment are well known to health professionals and are commonly referred to as "anorexic tricks."[13] Tricks enable persons with anorexia to conceal and cloak their real intention, losing weight. The purpose of tricks is to convince observers that nothing is untoward and they are fine. The art of "pulling tricks," as Michel de Certeau reminds us, is deployed by those in subordinate positions of power, takes advantage of opportunities, and mobilizes itself "in the service of deception." Trickery operates "within the enemy's field of vision [the enemy in this case being the staff], or the terrain imposed on it—it vigilantly makes use of cracks and is a guileful ruse" (1984, 37).[14] One therapist quoted by Bemis-Vitousek noted the variety of tricks that people diagnosed with anorexia pull on caregivers, in these cases in the form of lies: "Well, I don't eat meat for ethical reasons . . . I don't eat butter because it's bad for your health . . . I don't use vegetable oil because I don't like its slimy texture . . . I don't eat sugar because I'm allergic to it . . . I don't eat much at any one time because I hate to feel stuffed . . . I exercise three hours a day because it relieves tension. You are asking me why I lost 30 pounds? I didn't mean to, it just happened" (1997, 5).[15]

Other tricks include drinking liters of water or hiding bars of soap in underwear before being weighed and always taking the stairs instead of a lift or refusing to wear warm clothes in winter to burn more calories. These common tactics do not surprise professionals, but when an unusual trick comes to light, they may comment on it as ingenious, creative, or bizarre. During a ward round a young woman who was spitting her food out after chewing it was described by a clinician as "rather unusual"—despite a number of my participants telling me that they did this routinely.

The language of concealment became a therapeutic device in one eating-disorder unit, where the psychiatrists described the thinking that becomes engrained among diagnosed anorexics as "magical or superstitious." They suggested to patients that anorexia was magical, for it "masked" the person's thinking and actions and created the illusion of a distorted body image through trickery and deception. Anorexia and, by extension, the people with this diagnosis could not be trusted (see also Coopman 1995, 1).

The Distinction of Secrecy

As my fieldwork relationships with participants deepened over time, I became aware of the importance of concealment and secrecy to the logic of practice that underpinned anorexia. The power of secrecy lies not only in what it conceals—trying to hide practices from staff, friends, and family, for instance—but also in what it reveals and creates. Strathern and Herdt both argue that what is missing from the comparative study of secrecy is an understanding of how secret collectives, by creating social hierarchies, are systems that produce cultural meaning (Herdt 1990, 368; Strathern 1988, 115). Strathern highlights the ways in which secrecy in Gimi cultures enabled the actors to play the parts they allocated themselves, thus controlling their meaning. Such secrecy establishes an exclusive domain in which only certain sets of meanings have value; others were suppressed or rendered irrelevant (1988, 204).

In the case of my research, whether staff knew about tricks or secrets was in many ways immaterial, because it was the creation of meaning—what Estelle described as "the whole culture behind anorexia"—that gave people with anorexia exclusive relationships of power, knowledge, and practice. It was the performance of secrecy, rather than its content, that was productive.

Secrecy was a distinctive feature of anorexia and, as Taussig notes, where there is secrecy there is power (and vice versa) (1999, 7). The performance of secrecy enabled participants to hide anorexic practices and vehemently state that they "were fine" (see also Peters 1995, 44); it distinguished them from those with other illnesses, both medical and psychiatric; and when people came together in treatment settings it had the potential to establish a collective and new relationships through a common diagnosis and experiences. Some participants suggested that there was a "secret language of eating disorders" that was articulated through a range of bodily practices that were known and shared among those with anorexia. Although some chose not to engage with the collective secrecy, all knew of its existence and power from their own day-to-day strategies of concealment. These secret knowledges and practices were most clearly displayed when people participated in treatment programs, for it was here that the sense of belonging to the anorexic identity was most important and yet most at risk (from the threat that one's anorexia could be exposed and one thus disempowered). It was in these spaces that anorexic practices were challenged and confronted, yet these were the places where the hierarchy of anorexia was most evident, as some competed to be the best anorexic within the group.

Secrecy thus operated to mark differences between people within and outside anorexia and in doing so created status and prestige for those who practiced it. Those who maintained their anorexia described feeling a sense of superiority over everybody else they encountered. Anorexia was, particularly in the early phases of the experience, a productive and empowering state of distinction. It was not experienced as a debilitating illness, but as a state that was "unique," "heroic," "an achievement," "a thrill," "a high" in which people felt "indestructible" and "superhuman." Rita summed up the pride associated with anorexia: "When I was diagnosed with anorexia, I was secretly proud. One of the features of when you're extremely thin is bloody pride, you're bloody proud of yourself for getting down to skeletal proportions. 'Oh, I'm strong, I did it, just a bit more.' . . . It was my special secret."[16]

This power of anorexia came from immersion in a habitus that promotes a particular representation of the female body as desirable and valuable. Lynch argues that "in the weight-conscious West the human body is now the ultimate commodity," inextricably interwoven with the emphasis on thinness and success (1987, 128). The body has thus become a source of "symbolic power based on the possession of symbolic capital" (Bourdieu 1990, 138). In standing out above the crowd by excelling at its own rules, participants publicly and viscerally attested to the embodied distinction of symbolic power.

Unpacking Secrecy

Unpacking secrecy is an important first step in understanding the logic of anorexia, for it points to the ways in which secrecy operates to create exclusion, difference, and power for its keepers. Secrecy has many guises: its primary function is to conceal and hide, but "concepts of sacredness, intimacy, privacy, silence, desire, danger and deception all influence the way we think about secrecy" (Bok 1982, 26). These guises intertwine and sometimes conflict, but are all fundamental to the ways in which belonging is expressed, that is, to the ways in which the power of secret knowledges and practices are possessed and made use of.

Sisella Bok's *Secrets* explores how secrets have come to be known through language (stories, myths, and literature) and experience. Of secrecy she writes: "From earliest childhood we feel its mystery and attraction. We know both the power it confers and the burden it imposes. We learn how it can delight, give breathing space, and protect. But we come to understand its dangers, too: how it is used to oppress and exclude; what can befall those who come too close to secrets they were not meant to share; and the price of betrayal" (1982, xv).

Associations of privacy and intimacy with secrecy are particularly important, as they serve to compound many of the practices associated with anorexia. People vomit, for example, when they are sick, usually in private and seen as disgusting when not. Vomiting and purging intentionally, rather than as the consequence of a sickness, had to be kept secret, or one ran the risk of public shame and ridicule. In a similar way, the once public and communal activities of eating and exercising enter the private and intimate anorexic world. Both are done in secret; people with anorexia "often disguise the fact that they are eating at all, going to the refrigerator at night when no-one else can see them" (Claude-Pierre 1997, 183). This was why Natalia shopped for food far from where she lived; it maintained her secrecy and anonymity when to be exposed could mean shame, embarrassment, and guilt.

Recent interpretive ethnographic work has reexamined the meanings associated with secrecy (see also Crook 2007). Herdt (1990) and Luhrmann (1989a, b), among others, start by recognizing the important findings of earlier accounts (see, for example Bellman 1984; Shils 1956; Simmel 1950; and Wedgewood 1930). They then similarly define secrecy as "an intentional process of differentiating included persons and entities from those excluded, while simultaneously building solidarity among secret sharers" (Herdt 1990, 360). Such authors have, however, criticized these early analyses for their positioning within a structuralist/functionalist divide in which society is opposed to the individual, and pushed the analysis further in a number of ways.

The major critique of earlier works, and of Simmel's classic 1950 study in particular, concerns the autonomy of a secret society. The secret society for Simmel is a singular social order that leaves no room for an alternative understanding of the shifting, heterogenous, and contested nature of secrecy (or of societies). Moreover, within this schema, there is no understanding of the ontological processes for the people involved; they simply merge into the secret society. Simmel spoke of the "de-individuation of the person, [thus implying] a loss of self/personhood through a complete merging and commitment of the person into the collective" (Herdt 1990, 363). Herdt argues to the contrary, suggesting that Simmel's "clouded understanding" on this point is motivated by a "Western ontology regarding the rational and magical in secrecy" (364). Herdt cites Young's critical examination of myth in Malinowski, Leenhardt, and Levy-Bruhl as a useful parallel argument; in conceptualizing myth as a social experience, Young states that "mythic thought is affective rather than intellectual, a matter of moods rather than ideas," an experience that sees "mythic participation as unity" (1983, 14).

Similarly, as an embodied social experience, secrecy constitutes and transforms the person, as Luhrmann argues in her ethnography of the occult in contemporary England: "the most compelling aspect of secrecy in modern magic is the impact it can have upon an individual's experience" (1989a, 161). Secrecy thus operates not simply in a secret society, but in the transformative relationships in which individuals participate.

Following this line of thought, the second criticism of earlier analyses of secrecy recognizes the multiple layers of hierarchy that can occur within secret collectives. Internal or vertical hierarchy has been identified: "secret collectives assemble hierarchies [not only] between outsiders and insiders, [but also] between members of the collective itself. Power and resources are at issue" (Herdt 1990, 360).[17]

Finally, critics have targeted the ways in which secrecy has tended to be moralized. The secret, for Simmel, reflects the moral badness of a person. According to Herdt, persons conceal information to avoid censure or punishment (1990, 365); they must be lying, cheating, deceiving, or manipulating.

Hiding, subterfuge, and concealment have thus been seen as a "negative" dimension of a dynamic process of cultural production (364). Among my participants, Rita pointed out that anorexic practices made her feel like a criminal, hiding in the closet for twenty years. Hiding made her feel guilty, shameful, and deceitful—all compounding her sense of herself as a "bad person." To conceal, though, as we have seen, is simultaneously to construct or fabricate a parallel and possibly entirely different system of signs (ibid). All the time that Rita was concealing practices, managing to hide the fact that she hadn't eaten, she was also constructing a space where she felt "good"—superior to those who did eat. There is always an obverse side to the negative with anorexia, and it is the production of meaning "in the closet" that is of importance.

The Distinction of Secrecy

The complex dynamic of secrecy in this anorexic context includes the ways in which relationships were transformed through the secret collectives of anorexia, the internal hierarchy of groups, and the difficulty individuals had in leaving the intimate connections of anorexia. The data highlight the dynamic interrelationships of concealing and revealing that occurred with and between people who had a diagnosis of anorexia.

The Secret Collective

I knew that I could not always gain access to people's private and secret experiences, as I have mentioned. Monica, who used her own experiences of eating disorders in her therapy, suggested that whether or not I had experienced anorexia would greatly affect my research: "You sit with a group of people with eating disorders and they have their own language. If you haven't been there, you don't understand it." Participants were clear about when they were telling me a secret or letting me into an area of privileged knowledge.

Being "let in" recognizes a spatial separation. The insider/outsider dynamic was often characterized in spatial terms—those who were in or out of "the club." Sonya described the almost suburban and mundane inclusion: "I suppose I sort of see it as like an anorexic club—it's just like everyone is pretty accepting of you if you are sick, everyone's friends and stuff like that, and there's a bit of competition going on. It's sort of like you put in your membership and it's really hard to get out." I asked how one got into the club and who its members are. "It's sort of like a coffee club," she said. "You meet, you discuss the illness, . . . you have these friends—you're suddenly in this group and people understand you; . . . for me it was like my life had just been nothing for such a long time. That was all I knew, it was all I did, and I didn't have any outside life, and so suddenly I'm meeting all these people who don't have any sort of life either so it was just perfect. What else do we have to talk about? Nothing but anorexia."

Engaging with others who had the same diagnosis opened up new doors of relatedness for participants. They characterized having anorexia as if belonging to a persuasive and powerful group—"a religion," "a competitive sporting team," or part of "a game." Sonya explained that she was able to tell me things because she had "been a traitor and left the cult of anorexia." She stopped to explore her use of the word "cult": "I consider anorexia to be a secretive cult. . . . It's very much like a cult—you have to belong and there are certain things you don't share with the so-called normal people but you can share with each other. . . . It's a cult because anorexia brainwashes you, and if you don't cut the cord, it will kill you."

People with eating disorders group together and mark themselves as distinct from others. In hospital wards they formed cliques, sat together in the dining rooms, sat on each other's beds to swap stories, and maintained connections after their admissions. They separated themselves from those with other psychiatric disorders like schizophrenia. Amanda voiced an understanding common among those with anorexia that they are *extraordinary* rather than abnormal: "In many ways we're very normal. Like anorexia—okay it is a mental disorder, but it's not as debilitating as some of the others. For example, when I was under observation for two weeks, I was in a room with four beds and the girl next to me was—she was crazy. I don't mean that in a derogatory sense, but she'd have hallucinations and she had a tendency towards violence. . . . It was really scary; . . . myself and the other eating-disorder patients tried to avoid these people and you felt a bit sort of like, 'I'm not like these people, why have you put me in here?' I have a problem with food, but that's it—I'm not crazy."

Distinctions, or what participants called "battle lines," were also drawn against those who wanted to help them. "People [with anorexia] build such a wall around themselves," said Rita, "such a safety net of anorexia that anyone who comes along and tries to threaten that has got to be viewed as an enemy." The enemy included the doctors and nurses, who were seen as taking away the relationship people had with anorexia.[18] The kitchen staff were called the "kitchen witches" and pictured spreading lashings of butter onto sandwiches with the sole intention of fattening up the patients.

Undercover practices of resistance were in place, as we have seen, either solitary resistances or collective, organized attempts. These strategies of trickery were a form of *la perruque*—tactics of resistance that blended in with the surroundings, camouflaged so as not to draw attention to themselves, liable to disappear into their colonizing organization (de Certeau 1984, 31). Although de Certeau characterizes *la perruque* as operating in the workplace, that is by no means the only space in which this tactic occurs: "*La perruque* is infiltrating itself everywhere and becoming more and more common. It is only one case among all the practices which introduce *artistic* tricks and competitions of *accomplices*, . . . sly as a fox and twice as quick: there are countless ways of 'making do'" (29, emphasis in original).

Lacking their own space, participants made do within "a network of already established forces and representations" (de Certeau 1984,18). Vomiting and hiding food were difficult in patients' rooms because toilet and shower en suites were locked, and hand basins had the plumbing underneath removed so nothing could be disposed of or flushed away. People had to be ingenious in getting rid of food and vomit, and the more creative disposal schemes were trade secrets that they joked and laughed about—to perruque the system was to outwit the staff and to win. The staff knew about the common stashes of uneaten butter in people's shower bags or bins, but the butter scraped into duvet covers, under the metal lip of the side locker, or between the pages of a newspaper to be unwittingly taken home by a caring relative was divulged by participants in excited and hushed tones. When people were confronted by staff, they vehemently denied these practices, desperate to keep their secrets safe. There is, however, a simple glucose test that determines if the yellow fluid in a bedpan is in fact urine, or apple juice. Sometimes people gave in and admitted defeat, unable to provide excuses for the vomit squeezed into cosmetic containers or orange juice poured into flower vases.

Depending on the type of treatment program, some participants spent lengthy periods in single rooms. Here activity was reduced to moving on the bed; the only time they could leave the room was to be escorted and wheeled to the shower under a privilege system. Interaction with other patients was curtailed, but handwritten letters were secretly passed from one door to another, swapping stories of how to exercise without being noticed. And those who were allowed the freedom of the ward sometimes established cheating groups, banding together like a relay team.[19] Rita described how she was included in a network of food avoidance without warning—the fact that she had an eating disorder automatically meant she was an accomplice in a network of deception:

> We're a secretive lot; . . . this young girl tried to set up a little network of accomplices—like a support system to help her cheat. She even shoved a bag of nuts into my hand that was her supper. We were just walking past each other in the corridor and she shoved a bag of nuts in my hand and kept walking and . . . so I was actually aiding and abetting her by doing that. . . ., but I don't know why I didn't. I guess because you can see both sides and being older I can see the nurses' and doctors' perspective, but on the other hand I know how desperate she was to lose those nuts. She didn't want to put them in her body.

The secrecy that operated within the clinical setting not only propelled people with anorexia together, but also encouraged intimacy between them.

Some professionals recognized the double-edged nature of establishing or maintaining eating-disorder therapy groups, arguing that it provided a forum to fuel levels of competition and secrecy among those who already had strong bonds of intimacy. Several major hospitals had stopped running support groups altogether because they had the unintended effect of perpetuating eating-disorder practices. Staff who facilitated therapeutic groups and the community live-in program were well aware of the strong relationships that pivoted around anorexia and tried to encourage independence outside the safety and support of illness.

After leaving Lane Cove and the other treatment settings, people with anorexia continued friendships, with some even choosing to share apartments—a move that was firmly discouraged by staff. Those who went their separate ways often kept in touch by letter, e-mail, or phone, their relationships refracted through the commonality of eating disorders. Estelle, for example, kept in touch with a friend she made in the hospital whom she called "bulimia Ben." A group of nine women who had met in treatment at a private hospital had formed a competitive netball team named Chicken Legs that played weekly. In my local community when people spoke about those they knew with anorexia, I often already knew them because they had also participated in this research project. Several stories circulated among staff and patients had reached almost mythic proportions. Jacqui, for example, was well known within eating-disorder circles. She had had an eating disorder for most of her life and now in her forties was facing life-threatening complications as a result. During her multiple hospital admissions she had befriended many younger women and warned them of the consequences of their practices. Her struggle with anorexia was often evoked in ward rounds or in conversations I had with informants.

Secrecy was not only defined by treatment settings—those with anorexia were aware of a sense of possession and of cohesiveness that was not defined by a coming together. Simmel argues that secret societies tend to be conscious of themselves as a group (1950, 363). They have a shared predicament that binds them. This was certainly the case in public spaces such as gyms or shopping malls, where people would point out others who had anorexia. They were strangers, but they "just knew" who was "in" by their distinctive bodily comportment—"the dead look" in their eyes, the sallowness of their upper arms, and the heaviness of their gait. These bodily signs meant that people could easily distinguish between those who were "naturally thin" and those who were anorexic, as Beth commented:

> The first thing that always gets my attention is the arms—[the upper arms] because they look disproportionately thin; . . . and in

the face—there's a look in the eyes. People used to say it about me, and I could never see it in myself but I can recognize it in other people—their eyes are dead. And if you've known someone, it's particularly noticeable, and then you see them—like there's no life behind them, it's just emptiness. So I find the face and the eyes the biggest giveaway, but in terms of the body, the arms. It's something you recognize—like the haggard look, the dead eyes, and just a weariness; and I don't know whether it was having been through it—it touched something in me and I recognized it.

Recognition between anorexics was an invitation to form a relationship. It initiated an exchange of comforting words at a bus stop or across the plaza on the university campus, and at other times it allowed for comparisons and exchange of purging techniques. Other recognition cues related to food practices—the trade secrets of avoiding food and purging—and the more common ways of avoiding eating, such as claiming to be vegetarian for moral reasons, saying that you'd already eaten, excusing yourself to the toilet once too often, or pushing the food on your plate around to make it look less like a full serving. Anorexia was in itself a vehicle of communication and connection.

Climbing the Hierarchical Ladder

One function of secrecy was to distinguish members from outsiders. Within the group however, equality was not the only effect of boundary marking, for anorexia involved competition with oneself or others, and the game was very seductive. An example of this competition was played out in the scene that opened this book, when the extremely underweight Josie came to stay with the Lane Cove residents, where the seduction to compete was a risk to the slow process of recovery.

Many participants spoke about the insidious levels of competition in anorexia. Sonya likened anorexia to a highly competitive sporting event: "It's like the Olympics—whoever is the thinnest has won the gold medal. The ultimate goal is to be the sickest, and the ultimate victory is death. Everybody wants to be the Olympic winner—the worst case, the one who survived three heart attacks and a stroke and was in a coma for five weeks. . . . It's just like attaining that religious level in a cult of self-sacrifice. It's very rewarding in a sick way."

"The best," Amanda reiterated, "is dead—that's when you win. The best you can be being anorexic is when you die." In their exploration of death and constructions of femininity, Malson and Ussher similarly describe the perilous competition, quoting one of their interviewees: "I always wanted to be the perfect anorexic, but I know the perfect anorexic's a dead one basically" (1997, 57).

The path of the best anorexic was the "purest." People referred to "pure" or "true" anorexia: weight loss by total control through almost total abstinence from food and drink. Unlike the binge/purge anorexics, purists did not need the aid of laxatives or vomiting; their path had no crutches. Pure anorexia, or true ana, was an important way of distinguishing themselves not only from other people, but also from other eating disorders, which were seen as lower down the scale. Those who binged and vomited fell into the bulimic category and were disparaged for their messiness and weakness—their loss of control, their falling prey to the desire of appetite. "People with bulimia are totally out of control and disgusting because they binge and purge. They cheat—they don't go the hard slog like [we] do," said Briony. Compulsive eaters don't come anywhere near the mark and were disparaged for their outright gluttony.

In *Wasted*, Hornbacher vividly captures the competitive aspirations of those with anorexia:

> When I got to treatment the first time, I was not one of the emaciated ones. I was definitely slim, far thinner than is normal or attractive, but because I was not visibly sick, the very picture of sick, because I did not warrant the coveted title of Anorexic, I was embarrassed. Ignore the fact that my diastolic pressure had a habit of falling through the floor every time I stood up, putting me on watch for sudden cardiac arrest, or the fact that my heart puttered along, slow and uneven as an old man taking a solitary walk through the park. Ignore the fact that I had a perforated esophagus and a nasty habit of coughing blood all over my shirt. In treatment, as in the rest of the world, bulimia is seen as a step down from anorexia, both in terms of medical seriousness and in terms of admirability. Bulimia, of course, gives in to the temptations of the flesh, while anorexia is anointed, is a complete removal of the bearer from the material realm. Bulimia harkens back to the hedonistic Roman days of pleasure and feast, anorexia to the medieval age of bodily mortification and voluntary famine. In truth, bulimics do not usually bear the hallowed stigmata of a skeletal body. Their self torture is private, far more secret and guilty than is the visible statement of anorectics, whose whittled bodies are admired as the epitome of feminine beauty. There is nothing feminine, delicate, acclaimed, about sticking your fingers down your throat and spewing puke. (1999, 153)

This hierarchy of eating disorders was unwittingly replicated by health professionals, who commonly refer to the ABC of eating disorders—anorexia, bulimia, and compulsive eating (Grieves 1997, 78; Melville 1983). Some participants who were initially categorized as bulimic were told by their psychiatrist that they were "failed anorexics." They did not fulfill the requirements for a diagnosis of anorexia (their weight loss was not significant and they purged their bodies rather than abstaining from food) and were thus seen as unsuccessful in their goals. Rather than give the game away, which such a comment would hope to encourage, the words served only to compound a sense of disgust at their failure and spurred them on to greater heights of abstinence.[20]

Cutting the Cord

Leaving anorexia was not a straightforward process for participants. Because anorexia offered much support, both individually and collectively, it was difficult to cut the cord. Those who left were not considered well or healthy, but "outside anorexics," traitors, and frauds. Leaving meant, as Hornbacher writes, losing the communication and connectedness that practices of anorexia form between women: "when you decide to throw down your cards, push back from your chair, and leave the game, it's a very lonely moment. Women use their obsession with weight and food as a point of connection with one another, a commonality even between strangers. Instead of talking about why we use food and weight control as a means of handling emotional stress, we talk ad nauseam about the fact that we don't like our bodies" (1999, 283).

Leaving anorexia also meant severing an intimate connection with a friend that was part of, and in some instances central to, who people considered themselves to be. Elise, for example, started to call herself Ana (a common label for anorexia among participants), for not only did she have her family and doctors telling her she was anorexic, but also she felt that it was pivotal to her sense of identity: "I became Ana, not Elise." Whether people experienced Ana as part of or representative of who they were, it was always described as a most difficult relationship to cut.

Sitting with me in our usual seat in the park one day, Rita described the difficulty of "letting the eating disorder go." She had "a powerful dream" in which an image of a little girl "was walking away from me"—she paused—"it was leaving." Rita started to cry, describing the intense loss and sadness at the thought of having to say goodbye to her "little friend" (the eating disorder). She returned to this dream later in the afternoon and told me why it "moved" her so much:

> It was like I was losing someone, but in a way I think that little kid was not the little me but the little matey that I was attempting at that point in time to kick out. But there was an infinite sadness in seeing—the little girl was actually the binge and she was leaving [starts to cry]. It sounds like bloody Hollywood crap but the child image was looking over the shoulder and the eyes looking so terribly sad. Loss. That wasn't an image of me, it was something that I was losing. It would be good

> if I did lose that part of myself, but I was infinitely saddened to be losing it, and as it happened I didn't. The little comfort mates are still there; . . . you don't want to lose them, they become like your little mates. You need them and you almost embrace them and they're the things that you hug and cuddle rather than people, because they're always there for you and to lose them would be to lose everything.

Anorexia was more than symptomatology for Rita. She experienced it not as alien or unwelcome (as many psychiatric disorders can be), but as part of herself, as a person with whom she had a relationship.[21] Even though Rita had attempted suicide on several occasions and had been close to death with low weights, she equated the loss of anorexia with her own death: "It's like, if you leave me I'll die; . . . it's the little faithful, loyal matey that's always there when I need them and will never let me down but it's not a mean little friend. It's not a demon friend, although sometimes I feel pretty clawed up inside and quite—on a visceral level, you know, that sort of gut-wrenching agony. But it's there and it's always been there. I'll die if I lose it—either I'll die if my little mate isn't there or I'll have nothing."

The strength of this bond was described by a male psychiatrist at the Scottish Eating Disorders Interest Group meeting when addressing other clinicians, researchers, and family members. To emphasize the power and emotive relationship that people have with anorexia, he asked which audience members had children. He chose one woman and engaged in a role-play with her in which she acted as herself (the mother) and he as an inspector for the child and adolescent youth services. In an authoritative manner, he proclaimed that she was not fulfilling her duties as a mother and that he had come to take her children away where they could be cared for properly. He acknowledged that while she might love her children, she was obviously not coping, as she was constantly exhausted, tired, and often angry and had on several occasions been seen physically harming them. He had come to take her children away, right then and there. This scenario, the psychiatrist argued, was what people with anorexia often confront when they attend treatment. This bond of kinship is now being used as an analogy in the training of some therapists (see also Bemis-Vitousek 1997, 11)

As Rita suggested, though, there is much ambiguity to the relationship one has with anorexia. Many participants characterized anorexia as a best friend but also as an enemy, like being in an abusive relationship from which it seemed impossible to walk away. For their 1999 article "Anorexia Nervosa: Friend or Foe?" Serpell and colleagues asked patients with a diagnosis of anorexia to write two letters to "their anorexia nervosa," one addressing it as a friend, and the other addressing it as the enemy. While their discussion highlights the positive reinforcement that anorexia as a friend maintains, the authors overlook the ambiguous nature of this disorder. Anorexia in a relationship represents *both* friend and foe. Rita encapsulated the contradictory nature of her experiences: "It's empowering but also enslaving. You're an absolute bloody slave to it; . . . it's your friend and your enemy, you bet. Yes, it's like the devil with a smile. 'Come here, I'm going to help you, I've got a good way for you to cope,' and then he sticks the fork in."[22] Others described anorexia as like a marriage that began with "a honeymoon phase" but transformed over time into a destructive relationship.[23] The only way to escape was to divorce themselves from what they termed their "abusive lover."

In this chapter I have examined experiences of belonging in a variety of contexts—participants' homes, treatment settings, public spaces, and the Internet. In all these spaces issues of relatedness were central: feeling alienated and disconnected from families, friends, and bodies; longing to have a diagnosis of anorexia; viewing anorexia as a secret friend and abusive lover; the sharing of anorexic practices that engendered belonging in hospital settings; being an "outside anorexic"; and leaving the group and friendships of anorexia behind.

Anorexia was not just a clinical entity but was coproduced and mobilized by a variety of people, knowledges, and representations. On the one hand it was authored by others (by psychiatrists and health care workers as described in chapter 2), and on the other hand it was displaced by the actions of those who were given the diagnosis. As Strathern has shown in exploring the phenomenon for Melanesian culture, the agent, or acting subject, may thus be less a locus for relationships than a "pivot of relationships . . . one who *from his or her own vantage point acts with another's in mind.*" In this view "the object or outcome is their relationship, the effect of their interaction" to be transformed or replicated (Strathern 1988, 272, emphasis in original).

Anorexia was a central pivot of relatedness as well as a vehicle for relatedness itself. By entering into a relationship with anorexia people had the capacity to own and disown it, conceal and reveal it, and in the process, create different types of relatedness that confounded taken-for-granted avenues of connection. Participants were thus constantly struggling and strategizing within and between sets of social relations.

Participants described anorexia as a friend *and* an enemy, a source of support; in Rita's experience, it replaced intimate physical contact. Concealing this relationship from those who would not understand the desires and motivations of anorexia was mandatory, and people went to great lengths to hide or deny anorexic practices. The shame of being exposed and the desire to continue a relationship with anorexia ensured secrecy. By avoiding social engagements of intimacy and commensality, participants radically altered social relations with those around them.

When participants entered treatment programs and met others with similar diagnoses, they learned of the secret collective surrounding anorexia. This collective was dynamic and changing, its boundaries always moving. Although practices were often revealed to other members of the group and close ties of affection and allegiance developed, there were those like Estelle and Rita who wanted to disconnect from this group and move away. No matter where people were positioned, they were aware of the relationships that anorexia provided and excluded.

5

Abject Relations with Food

> Loathing an item of food, a piece of filth, waste or dung. The spasms and vomiting that protect me. The repugnance, the retching that thrusts me to the side and turns me away from defilement, sewage, muck. The shame of the compromise, of being in the middle of treachery.
>
> —Julia Kristeva, *Powers of Horror*

A different field of relatedness—that between participants and food—now becomes my focus. The relationships that those diagnosed as anorexic have with food are often assumed to be an extension of taken-for-granted concepts around nutrition, concepts that are transformed into idiosyncratic routines aimed at weight loss. My research challenges this common assumption, exploring the various meanings that participants attributed to particular foods, and the practices involved. We see that food practices were central to the relationships that people with anorexia had with each other, their own bodies, and other people.

Here, I first discuss the genealogy of nutrition to show the ways in which nutrition has emerged in a variety of fields that influence people's everyday experiences and practices surrounding food. Nutrition, as many have argued before me, did not appear out of thin air. Next, I outline how participants' embodied responses to foods pointed my analysis toward Kristeva's visceral model of abjection. Finally, I extend Kristeva's psychoanalytic/literary concept of abjection to participants' everyday practices and relationships.

"You are what you eat": Nutritional Pedagogy

Each field that I encountered in my fieldwork shared a common currency of language about food and nutrition. In the medical realm, for example, food practices and habits were framed by biomedical explanations: anorexia was refracted through a discourse that took the disorder to be an extreme conformity to contemporary dietary regimes. Within this framework the physiological effects of not eating (effects of malnutrition such as osteoporosis or infertility) were of prime importance.

Dietitians were integral to redressing this imbalance and restoring a person's nutritional status. All medical teams had a dietitian on board, measuring people's weight and body mass index and calculating caloric diets that worked toward a target weight goal. They prescribed what foods all clients should eat, and at what times, and in what quantities. Khare similarly discusses how the nutritionist is interested in "prescription as well as description, gathering data to construct universals of the human diet and to pronounce on the appropriate foods, evincing a 'utopian' idea of the 'perfect human diet' to achieve perfect health" (Khare 1980, 526–527, cited in Lupton 1996, 7).

Even though my fieldwork traversed a variety of treatment settings, I found the authority of nutritional information taken for granted in each. At a private hospital I sat on Olivia's bed while she showed me how she planned her daily meals. Rather than by calories, the meal plan was categorized according to portions, with a "protein/carbohydrate exchange" system used to monitor intake. This form of treatment, while promoted as a radical alternative to mainstream services, works within a nutritional framework that uses the language and assumptions of that discourse.

The privileged status of nutritional discourse is the consequence of the history of nutritional science, in which the relationship between nutritional practices and wider discourses has been integrally connected. Although the concept of dietary regimens can be traced back to Hippocrates (based on a humoral system of health), nutrition as a science did not receive popular circulation until the late eighteenth century (Lupton 1996, 69). It is this period and onward that is of interest, for it here that the nutritional value of food (based on its chemical composition) emerged to combine with doctrines of good health, hygiene, and manners.

The history of nutrition, like all histories, is a contested one. In reviewing this contestation, Coveney (1999, 2006) argues that the debates have not allowed for a full appreciation of the heritage of ideas that are part of nutrition discourse. In particular, he points to the false separation of moral asceticism and scientific discoveries, as argued by Turner (1982) and Aronson (1982a) respectively. Turner suggests that the eighteenth-century English physician Cheyne, who wrote widely about the importance of dietary asceticism for health, was central to the development of Western discourses on diet (Coveney 1999, 23). Cheyne drew on a mechanical metaphor of the body, constructing it as "a complex series of pumps, pipes and canals [that could only be] maintained by the correct input of food and liquid, appropriate exercise and careful evacuation" (B. Turner 1982, 260). In a series of popular books published between 1724 and 1742, Cheyne theorized that a rich diet—"the rarest delicacies, the richest foods, and the most generous wines"—caused illness among "the Rich, the Lazy, the Luxurious, and the Unactive, those who fare daintily and live voluptuously" (Turner 1982, 261, cited in Lupton 1996, 70).

Cheyne's work had affinities with other areas of asceticism, particularly religious asceticism. Turner believes that John Wesley, the founder of Methodism, was directly influenced by the dietary asceticism promoted by Cheyne, not a surprising link considering the familiar spiritual practice of disciplining the body and purifying the soul through strict dietary practices.[1]

In contrast to Turner's rendering of nutritional history, Aronson argues that nutrition emerged in the late eighteenth and early nineteenth centuries through scientific knowledge of organic chemistry and its application to physiology (Coveney 1999, 23–24). She suggests that the origins of rationalization of the modern diet were located not in Cheyne's ascetic dietary regimes but in calculations about the food needs of different groups of people, of how the body converted food into energy (Aronson 1982b, 54). In this discourse, the body was seen as "a thermodynamic system in which food constituents provided energy for caloric output as work" (Coveney 1999, 24). Institutional populations in jails, armies, and workhouses were researched to provide evidence about various manual labors, occupations, and lifestyles and the corresponding dietary requirements.

Despite the cogency of each argument, Coveney suggests that these positions are two sides of the same system of thought: "The concern with the moral order has been, and indeed continues to be, central to and intimately bound with scientific enterprise" (1999, 24–25). The false separation of asceticism and science, he goes on to argue, has come about by locating the discovery of nutrition in the hands of bright physicians or scientists, as Turner and Aronson have done. Rather, nutritional science was "produced at a time when a range of population sciences such as social statistics, social sciences and population medicine informed the regulation of the law, poverty, health, life and conduct of individuals through the normalization of mundane activities." In Coveney's Foucauldian analysis, nutrition developed amid a number of historical developments and social procedures, rather than individual lives. These developments, which came to fruition in the nineteenth century, were "part of a panoply of technologies and strategies designed to better manage populations" (2000, xi).[2]

Coveney notes that dietary guidelines for populations, initially developed in the United States in the 1970s, have now been developed for nearly all countries in the industrialized world: "Although differing slightly in content, these guidelines spell out dietary goals for each county's population, for example, "eat less fat," "eat more fruit and vegetables," "eat less sugar," "eat less salt" and so on" (1999, 23; see also Coveney 2008).

Even this very brief overview of the history of nutritional science reflects an increasing concern for the governing of people's diets. This regimentation, in Foucault's terms, has meant increased surveillance, rationalization, and regulation of what people eat, all supported and authenticated by scientific claims and knowledge of the medical field. Diet has become a highly visible aspect of people's lives that should be regulated in the interests of good health.[3] It has also become a moral question, "involving issues of an individual's capacity for self-control and work and the avoidance of waste and excess" (Lupton 1996, 73). Coveney sums up this convergence of institutional structure and everyday practice:

> On the one hand there was a government of others [populations] through the development of food classifications, registers and recommended allowances against which food habits could be scientifically assessed, complete with the survey as an instrument of "the Panopticon" (Foucault's "technologies of power"). On the other hand, through the imperative to eat "properly," nutrition was constructed as a moral choice where individuals were required to be ethical; to problematize their food choices, consider their actions, thoughts and desires in hopes of becoming "good," rational, healthy subjects (Foucault's "technologies of the self"). (Coveney 1999, 33)

The salience of these nutritional ideas, of scientific evidence and moral imperatives, is readily available in the public domain. It is taken for granted that most people have had some level of engagement with these nutritional ideas through schools, family environments, public health campaigns, children's centers, local health practitioners, the media, and even packets of supermarket food. One participant learned of the moral values and dangers of cholesterol and fats through her mother's work at the Heart Foundation. Maddy had ready access to the health promotional literature that outlined the "good and bad fats," including the suggested daily intake and the effects of too much fat on one's body and overall health.[4] Armed with this knowledge, she limited herself to three thousand kilojoules a day (239 calories)—fats were blacklisted—and in a scientifically rigorous manner she meticulously measured and recorded her daily oral intake.

Conforming to orthodox nutritional advice, people seek to control their diet to achieve good health rather than eating foods that they may prefer because of taste. The very notion of nutrition, Lupton suggests, "is a functionally orientated one: food is for nourishing, for fuelling the body, for building bones, teeth and muscle, a means to an end. Food preferences, tastes and habits are considered secondary to what food does biologically to the body" (1996, 7). This stripping away of the sociocultural context of nutrition was promoted by some health professionals I encountered in my fieldwork. A psychiatric nurse, for example, responded to Angela's anxiety about and fear of foods that she was presented with on a weight-gain program by suggesting that she think of food as "just a fuel. It's just a fuel to keep the body running, nothing more."

The relationship between nutritional status, health, and food consumption can be reproduced with ease. In her analysis of the relationship between food, embodiment, and subjectivity, Lupton asked participants in her focus groups and interviews to describe "unhealthy foods" and found that "almost all of them nominated fatty or 'greasy' foods, junk or fast food, salty foods, fatty red meat, chocolate, soft drinks and other sugary foods. Foods described as 'healthy' were typically vegetables and fruit (particularly if 'fresh'), salads, whole grains, lean meat, chicken and fish" (1996, 81).

These ideas of healthy and nonhealthy foods were clearly used by participants in my project. Beth showed me her lists of bad foods and good foods.[5] The bad food list, which was more than twice the length of the other, had "fried" as the first listed food: this included fried bacon, egg, chips, and rice. After this, foods high in fat content were marked (cheeses, pizza, biscuits, and red meats), followed by processed foods and those high in sugars and complex carbohydrates. The good food list included most vegetables and fruits (excluding pears and potatoes), low-fat yoghurts, high-calcium/low-fat milk, and skinless chicken.

The public spaces mentioned earlier, from child care services to general practice waiting areas, have a poster exhibiting the "Five Food Groups Pyramid"—a hierarchical arrangement with the bad foods at the top (fats and oils) and the good foods at the bottom (vegetables and cereals). Participants were conversant with this model, often telling me about the pyramid in conversations about food. When Elise left the hospital program, she confided in me that she had reverted to eating only from the bottom of the pyramid: fruit, vegetables, rice, cereal, low-fat milk, and diet yoghurt.

As the historical outline of nutritional discourse reveals, ideas of healthy food are constantly changing. The most recent change in nutritional education (which occurred during my fieldwork) has been the replacement of the triangular model with a circular one. It was via the Eating Disorder Association newsletter that I learned of this change and saw the new representation of healthy eating. Although the visual hierarchy has gone, five food groups remain, yet the once included unhealthy category of fats and oils is relegated to the corner of the image with the advice to "choose these sometimes in small amounts." In many ways, fats and oils have been marginalized even further from daily consumption. This diagram does not consider fat a valuable component of food consumption. Despite the distinction of good from bad fats (of polyunsaturated from saturated), contemporary nutritional, medical, and popular discourses continue to represent fat as unhealthy, bad, and unnecessary.

Why have fats been further marginalized from daily food consumption? At the most basic level, it is the literal translation of the word "fat": if one consumes fatty foods, then one will become fat. As the moralistic dietary message reminds us, "We are what we eat." Dietary messages constantly tell us to reduce our fat intake, and if one consumes more than the daily requirement of fat, one will become fat.[6] For people with a diagnosis of anorexia, "fat" literally translates into a physical and emotional feeling, as Estelle explained: "We don't say,'Oh, I feel a bit sugary today' but will often say, 'I feel fat' or 'I am fat.'" Estelle further explained why she able to eat sugar but not fat:

> I guess it's because sugar dissolves. It's not such a solid thing, do you know what I mean? You get sugar in a soft drink or something and it doesn't leave the same sort of greasy or heavy feeling either, and you can see fat, whereas sugar—I suppose I got the image of sugar dissolving into my system and going into my muscles and being burnt off like that, whereas I had the image of the fat sort of just sitting in my stomach. You think of this stuff here [pinches her stomach] and you think of that as fat, not sugar. . . . Like everyone says, "You're fat," not "[You're] sugar." . . . I feel fat because I ate fat. . . . I could almost imagine it just going straight onto my thighs, or my bum, or my tummy, whereas the sugar I imagine diluting through my system.

When Fat Is Not Fat

People with anorexia clearly used the rhetorical devices of fear of fat that are current in popular and nutritional discourses. But I found that there were additional meanings of food and fat unavailable to those who did not belong to anorexia.

In his discussion on the role of embodied metaphor, Kirmayer highlights the ways in which people attribute entirely different meanings to the same seemingly neutral "facts." He outlines the case of Mr. Y, a thirty-five-year-old businessman receiving hemodialysis for chronic renal failure. The doctors wanted Mr. Y to have a blood transfusion to correct his dangerously low hemoglobin levels, but he refused. The reasons he gave for his refusal concerned ideas of contamination, as he was "terrified of receiving other people's blood because it may contain genetic material that carries their personality traits." The doctors considered this rationale absurd, as blood—in the biomedical domain—does not "contain genetic material . . . and genes do not transmit personality from one adult to another." Mr. Y understood the blood transfusion as threatening his bodily boundaries, of transgressing and polluting his body. "Blood" for the patient was not "blood" for the physician (1992, 325).

Kirmayer is drawing the reader's attention to the assumed universality of the meanings of medical language. Within biomedicine, the facts of biology are a given, and patients who hold differing beliefs may be, as in the case of Mr. Y, referred to a psychiatrist. Differing viewpoints are seen as false beliefs, misapprehensions, or "some hidden perversity of the patient's mind" (1992, 326).

I found a similar assumption at work among health professionals in relation to concepts of food and fat. During ward rounds it was assumed that factors contributing to an eating disorder were generally located in one's upbringing—one's sexual history, family relationships—and one's inability to cope with these. Very little space was given to participants' experiences of their bodies and relatedness outside this framework. There was, for example, no investigation of a young Jewish girl's beliefs surrounding the dietary law of her religion.[7] When I asked the treating psychiatrist if her beliefs might have a connection to the way she experienced anorexia, he replied: "It has nothing to do with her anorexia." Another woman had traveled extensively and lived in Japan, where she consulted a Japanese herbalist about her dietary concerns. Her "mystical ideas about food" and the belief that "her internal organs were twisted, sick, and out of place" were pathologized as a somatic illness or schizophrenia. She was described in the ward round as "quite mad," "not run of the mill," and "quite an unusual one."

How people with eating disorders view food is not central or problematic for health professionals. It is assumed that they take everyday, commonsense dietary guidelines to the extreme, to the point where they are no longer commonsense and hence "manifestations of individual pathology, of dysfunctional beliefs or faulty cognitions" (Malson 1998, 128). Yet as Geertz (1973) and Herzfeld (2001) have highlighted, common sense is itself a cultural system: "If common sense is as much an interpretation of the immediacies of experience, a gloss on them, as are myth, painting, epistemology, or whatever, then it is, like them, historically constructed and, like them, subjected to historically defined standards of judgement" (Geertz 1973, 76).

Anorexia is commonly referred to as "the slimmer's disease," a diet that has just gone too far. The current diagnostic definition assumes that people with eating disorders are afraid of becoming fat, and as a consequence, actively avoid fatty food (American Psychiatric Association 1994, 2000; World Health Organization 1992).[8] Although there are slightly different criteria in each definition, each includes references to the "fear of gaining weight or becoming fat," "feeling fat" and "the avoidance of fattening foods."[9]

But like Mr. Y, people with anorexia can have quite different beliefs about the nature of food and fat. "Food," like "blood," is not always "food" for the patient. It was not until I was four months into my fieldwork that I became aware of the varying meanings associated with foods. I too had assumed that people with anorexia have a fear of fat and of high-calorie foods and therefore avoid them. This was certainly how many people (including those diagnosed and health professionals) talked about anorexia, but there were a number of other meanings also at play. For a large number of participants, food was not life giving, it was life threatening. It was characterized as disgusting, polluting, contaminating, evil, poisonous, dirty, defiling, and harmful. Fats (butter,

margarine, and oils), in particular, were the most dangerous—not simply because of their fat content, but because of their form, their ability to move and seep into the cracks of one's body. It was these properties of food and fat that participants intensely feared, far beyond their concern with weight gain per se.

Food as "Matter out of Place"

Throughout my fieldwork I had been asking people how they experienced food, and what different foods meant to them. Commonsense dietary laws were easily articulated, and there were times when I thought no other meanings of food were operating, until a casual response highlighted a new way of understanding and experiencing food. Rita alerted me to a different framework around foods that not only drew on current nutritional advice but also had its own language, meanings, and practices. She assured me that these beliefs were part of the "manual of eating disorders" and that most members of "the club" would share the same understanding. She was surprised that she was the first to explain this to me, suggesting that it was central to many people's experiences of anorexia.

On reflection, I believe that part of participants' hesitancy in describing the hidden meanings of food and fats was related to the overall secrecy of some anorexic practices. The perception among those with anorexia was that others perceived these beliefs (and what was done to counter them) to be "very unusual," "weird," and "strange." These beliefs were described to me only when my relationship with a participant was well established, often through casual remarks or practices. They were almost exclusively couched in terms of embarrassment and irrationality.

In many ways, though, I should not be surprised at the time it took for people to share this understanding with me. Stoller (1997) describes any fieldwork situation as like an apprenticeship, where people choose to invite the ethnographer at different times to learn new meanings and understandings about certain events or practices. When I entered the field, I was at the ready for the unfamiliar, but it was attending to what was most familiar that provided me with an entrée into a whole new belief system around food. It was through embodiment—the sensory, the visceral, and the unspoken—that I began to learn of different levels of meaning. What initially obscured my understanding of how people with anorexia experienced food was my own assumption that we were sharing the same meanings of language and visceral responses to food.

Rita and I would often go in the afternoons to a public park not far from her house. We'd meet in the car park and then walk to a nearby wooden seat that overlooked a large pond and the grounds of the park. Being an animal lover, Rita once brought a loaf of white bread to feed the ducks as we sat and

chatted. We both broke the bread into small pieces and threw it to the ever-increasing number of expectant ducks. When it looked as if the ducks were losing interest, Rita closed the opening to the plastic bag of bread, turned on the seat, and looked earnestly around the park. I asked her what she was looking for and she replied: "I'm looking for a tap or a toilet block to wash my hands." "Why do you need to wash your hands?" I asked. "Oh," she said, quite matter of factly, "because they're dirty. I've touched food." This was the first time I had twigged to the correlation between food and dirt, and I could not overlook this response to food. Rita told me that she always washes her hands after she touches food, most particularly foods that are greasy and slimy, such as oils, butters, and uncooked meat. She also described a hierarchy of foods that was not necessarily predicated on the food pyramid or calorie or fat content. It was a hierarchy of clean and dirty foods: "Vegetables are okay to touch—they are clean and pure— whereas other foods, and the greasy ones in particular, are defiling, disgusting . . . polluting and contaminating. . . . You pollute your body by ingesting this stuff called food. . . . I find putting food in my mouth repugnant."

I returned to my field sites with a new focus. Many participants nodded knowingly and enthusiastically when I asked about "dirty foods," one woman telling me that I had now come a long way in my understanding of eating disorders. In reflecting on her experiences, Trudy sent me an e-mail: "Much of my anorexia was about being clean versus dirty. Not eating was clean. Eating was dirty, contaminating. It was not about being fat or thin. Nor was it about weight."

Looking back over my earlier field notes, I could now see these themes of purity and dirt circulating in people's narratives. My first informant, Sonya, had similarly described her wish to not eat in order to be "empty and clean. . . . I felt dirty when I ate. I still do sometimes, sort of grimy." Despite some idiosyncratic changes to their food lists (some, unlike Rita, viewed bread as clean), for all participants, fats, oils, butters, and meat (particularly red meat) came under the rubric "dirty."

Surprisingly, few authors (including those writing autobiographical works) have explored at any length the ways in which food is talked about and experienced by people with anorexia. Even though Malson, for example, reported that her informants viewed food as "dangerous, dirty, and disgusting," she explains food within a broader discourse of mind/body control (1998, 126). She suggests that food has become an object in dualist discourse, where "body management becomes central to the maintenance of self-integrity, and eating becomes an occasion when the body, something that is not me, 'takes over' and triumphs in the discursively produced conflict between mind/self and body" (125).

Bordo similarly describes the triumph of the will over the body: "One woman describes how after eating sugar she felt 'polluted, disgusting, sticky

through the arms, as if something bad had gotten inside me.'" Rather than exploring the particularities of language and embodiment, Bordo draws on a religious framework to explain this "tainting of the flesh" (1988, 95).

Malson, Bordo, and others (Hepworth 1999) talk about food almost generically, using either a gloss for all foods or an extension of nutritional education, good and bad foods, indulgent and dietary foods. There is no discussion of the distinction between foods.[10] When, on occasion, the embodied sensations of food are mentioned, they are overlooked or subsumed into disembodied discourses. What is lacking from the literature is an exploration of which foods in particular are defiling, and why some foods are more polluting than others. How do certain foods become dirty?[11]

Douglas's Typology: Dirt, Pollution, and Danger

In *Powers of Horror: An Essay on Abjection*, Kristeva suggests that "the logic of prohibition, which founds the abject, has been outlined and made explicit by a number of anthropologists concerned with defilement and its sacred function in so-called primitive societies" (1982, 64). Of these anthropologists it is Mary Douglas to whom Kristeva is most indebted, in particular her concepts of dirt and classification. Although Kristeva criticizes Douglas's classificatory schemes, they have much in common with Kristeva's psychoanalytic theory of abjection and emergent subjectivity and cannot be described without this acknowledgment.

Participants' use of the words "dirty" and "clean" was akin to Douglas's formulation of these terms. In *Purity and Danger* (1984) and *Implicit Meanings: Essays in Anthropology* (1975), Douglas describes how the concept of dirt emerges from a culture's classificatory system of order. It is at the margins or boundaries of these systems, though, that categories are most threatened and vulnerable. Some people, materials, events, or behaviors do not fit easily into these bounded categories and may be entirely ambiguous in their positioning. Douglas categorizes as out of place things that "blur, smudge, contradict, or otherwise confuse classifications" (1975, 51), and what is out of place, she argues, threatens the social order and is labeled dirty, dangerous, and polluting (see also Wood 1997, 28–29).

One of Douglas's classic examples of purity and danger relates to Jewish dietary law and the prohibition of certain foods laid down in the Old Testament book of Leviticus. In her chapter "The Abominations of Leviticus," Douglas asks: "Why should the camel, the hare and the rock badger be unclean? Why should some locusts, but not all, be unclean? Why should the frog be clean and the mouse and the hippopotamus unclean? What have chameleons, moles and crocodiles got in common that they should be listed together?" (1984, 41).[12]

She answers these questions by applying her theory of dirt, marginality, and pollution. Only animals who "fully conform to their class," such as birds that fly, fish that have fins and scales, and animals that walk on all four feet, chew their cud, and have cloven hooves are considered clean. Pigs were forbidden to Hebrews because they were creatures considered anomalous under this system of classification; pigs (and camels) are cloven footed but are not ruminants and this, Douglas argues, is the only reason given in the Old Testament for avoiding them (55; see also Grosz 1989, 75). Their positioning was ambiguous and therefore impure or polluting (Caplan 1994, 7).

Similarly, creatures that cross the boundaries of habitat through indeterminate forms of movement such as creeping, crawling, or swarming are "explicitly contrary to holiness" (Douglas, 56). The snake, for example, which slithers indeterminately on land or in the water, does not adhere to rigid categories and is therefore unclean, dangerous, and not fit for consumption.

Douglas applies this classification of boundaries to the body, which, she argues, is a model that can stand for any bounded system: "Its boundaries can represent any boundaries which are threatened or precarious. The body is a complex structure. The functions of its different parts and their relation afford a source of symbols for other complex structures. We cannot possibly interpret rituals concerning excreta, breast milk, saliva and the rest unless we are prepared to see in the body a symbol of society, and to see the powers and dangers credited to social structure reproduced in small on the human body" (115). The body thus becomes a metaphor that is used "in different ways to reflect and enhance each person's experience of society" (Douglas 1973, 16).

As with any bounded system, according to Douglas, the body is most vulnerable at its margins (the skin) and external openings/orifices (for example, the mouth, nose, or vagina): "all margins are dangerous; . . . any structure of ideas is vulnerable at its margins. We should expect the orifices of the body to symbolize its specially vulnerable points. Matter issuing from them [the orifices of the body] is marginal stuff of the most obvious kind. Spittle, blood, milk, urine, feces or tears by simply issuing forth have traversed the boundary of the body" (1984, 121).

Like food, sexual fluids have a liminal status in terms of the permeability of the human body, for they cross its boundaries. Of the bodily fluids, Douglas argues, the ones that are related to bodily functions of digestion and procreation (for Douglas and Kristeva this is menstrual blood rather than semen) are the most defiling (125).

Dirt or filth in Douglas's terms is not an inherent quality but applies to a boundary and, more particularly, "represents the object being jettisoned out of that boundary, its other side, a margin" (Kristeva 1982, 69). Danger arises "from failure to control the quality of what [the body] absorbs through the orifices; fear of poisoning, protection of boundaries, aversion to bodily waste products" (Douglas 1973, 16).

Douglas's concepts of dirt, danger, and pollution are particularly apt for our purposes in terms of participants' fear of certain foods. Participants described contact with food as a dangerous liaison, as it was a polluting substance that crossed bodily boundaries. Several attributed to food the properties of a contagious disease; it was "out of bounds" and to be avoided "like the plague." Many described the very act of eating—of food passing into the interior of the body—as contaminating and polluting. Rita described bringing food to her lips and into her mouth as "utterly repugnant," as it marked the passing of a pollutant (food) into her body: "I don't like anything on my lips. It's a sensation which I really don't like; . . . I've never worn lipstick for that reason. You see, when you eat, you actually try to make as little contact with your mouth as possible. You actually put the food directly in without touching the lips—that's the aim—chew and swallow and the whole operation needs to be awfully quick."[13]

Her lips were the gatekeepers to her mouth, "an interesting piece of facial equipment" that Rita described as "a soft, moist, and sensitive area." Once inside the mouth, food had contaminated her body. It had crossed from "the external into the internal world; . . . it's inside you, it has been imbibed and internalized and there is a sense of feeling dirty and impregnated with something."

Skin contact with food was also problematic, as Rita's earlier account of touching bread demonstrated. Beth said that the only way she could explain her abhorrence of touching food was by describing something to me that "would make your body retch": "I felt dirty in regards to all food I ate. I felt contaminated, for want of a better word. I only felt pure when I was empty." I asked for clarification: "When you say contaminated, what do you mean?" She said: "Like [pauses] impure and sort of sullied. . . . I'll try and describe it. You know how, just say if you're sitting on the grass outside and you turn around and put your hand in dog poo, it's that sort of feeling, that sort of contamination. . . . So you don't want to prepare food—well, I wouldn't anyway, but you don't touch anything." Beth's equation of food with excreta was echoed by other participants. They described food, and fats in particular, as "dirt," "filth," "junk," "rubbish" and "shit."[14]

Because of their ambiguity within Douglas's classificatory system, foods that move (like fats and oils) are potentially dangerous and polluting. Moreover, in this schema food is doubly defiling because it passes through the oral boundary of the mouth, thereby transgressing the boundaries and margins of bodily order. Once inside the body, food mixes with saliva, travels through the alimentary system, and is transformed into an unrecognizable substance through digestion. When I asked Rita to describe the polluting or contamination of food, she captured the horror of digestive transformation: "It's like injecting or introducing—you might as well be drinking thick, gunky, sticky glue—that's the image of ingestion: sticky, and gunky, and slidy, and slimy. It turns into all of that as it goes through—it turns into gunk. Because I'm bulimic now and I'm bingeing, I see food as not only in and of itself junk and gunk and rubbish that I'm imbibing and therefore becomes even worse. It makes me fat and it's like I'm loaded up with—it's like I'm a balloon of glue or something, an ugly bag of gunk, . . . and it's so much better to not eat. It's much better to abstain." Digestion and decomposition move food from one category to another, from food to waste.[15]

While Douglas provides many insights into participants' experiences of food, this research also highlights the limitations of her theory. This is not to say that Douglas is outmoded or irrelevant; far from it. My critique of her work, which is in line with that of numerous others, has made possible a trajectory of ideas concerned with embodiment, particularly with the relational and sentient aspects of embodiment.

The main critiques of Douglas's work form part of a broader critique of the structuralist genre of anthropological theory. Her work is clearly informed by the intellectual legacies of sociological and anthropological theorists, of Durkheim, Mauss, and Lévi-Strauss. The general theme of Douglas's work is the relationship between the social and physical body, in that the social body constrains how the physical body is perceived and experienced (Shilling 1993, 73). Thus, as she argues in *Natural Symbols* (1973), the human body is the most readily available image of a social system; it is a metaphor for society as a whole. These theories are "sociocentric," in that Douglas "has her eyes uncompromisingly fixed on society as such" (Strathern 1996, 15).[16]

Emphasis on a social body results in a body that is profoundly disembodied, far removed from the phenomenological worlds of lived experience and practice. In Douglas's formulation (and Malson's and Bordo's preceding accounts), lived bodies are reduced to positions and categories made available by the broader social body. Moreover, her two bodies—the social and physical—reiterate the distinctions between mind and body, culture and biology. Within this formulation the individual body continues to reproduce these Cartesian binaries of a contained, rational unit that has distinct boundaries of inside/outside. The ontology that is at the very heart of structuralist thinking has been heavily critiqued, for it configures the body as representational: as fixed, ahistorical, prescriptive, and universal (see also Leder 1990; Csordas 1994).[17]

Understanding Abjection

Although relying heavily on Douglas's concepts of dirt and pollution, Kristeva distanced herself from what she called the "structural-functional X-ray of defilement": "As a matter of fact, the explanation she [Douglas] gives of defilement assigns in turn different statuses to the human body: as ultimate cause of the socio-economic causality, or simply as metaphor of that socio-symbolic being constituted by the human universe always present in itself. In so doing, however, Mary Douglas introduces willy-nilly the possibility of a subjective dimension within anthropological thought on religions. Where then lies the subjective value of these demarcations, exclusions, and prohibitions that establish the social organism as a 'symbolic system'?" (Kristeva 1982, 69, 66). In *Powers of Horror* (1982), Kristeva shifted Douglas's focus from the social body to the lived experience of gendered bodies (in this case female) and redirected the analyses from structuralism to psychoanalysis, from semantics to subjectivity. It was, as I argue further on, a shift from one extreme to another.

Abjection is a somewhat slippery concept to define, for it has multiple dimensions and is capable of various interpretations. The word "abject" literally means to cast off, exclude, or prohibit, yet abjection is defined by its relationship to desire—"like an inescapable boomerang, [it is a] vortex of summons and repulsion[s]" (Kristeva 1982, 1).[18] Even so, it seems impossible to pin down abjection, for, as Kristeva writes: "When I am beset by abjection, the twisted braid of affects and thoughts I call by such a name does not have, properly speaking, a definable *object*. The abject is not an object facing me, which I name or imagine. . . . The abject has only one quality of the object—that of being opposed to I" (ibid., emphasis in original).

"Abject" and "abjection" thus refer not only to a "sensation and attitude," but to that which is expelled "as well as to the act of throwing it away" (Grosz 1990, 87; Ellman 1990, 181). "Abjection" also refers to a space between the preoedipal and the oedipal of simultaneous pleasure and danger, of repulsion and attraction. As neither subject nor object, abjection is "an unnameable, pre-oppositional, permeable barrier that requires some mode of control or exclusion to keep it at a safe distance from the symbolic and its orderly proceedings" (Grosz 1990, 93).

Kristeva's psychoanalytic theory of abjection is concerned with an individual's process of self-identification. She claims that this process occurs in the early years of life when a child gains identity and a place within the symbolic order by separating from its mother. Abjection thus testifies to a break in the mother-child dynamic where the territorialization of space is enacted. It is the space of struggle against the mother, the "earliest attempts to release the hold of *maternal* entity even before ex-isting outside of her . . . It is a violent, clumsy breaking away, with the constant risk of falling back under the sway of a power as securing as it is stifling" (Kristeva 1982, 13, emphasis in original).

Symbolic language, Kristeva argues, is central to this break, for subjectivity has its genesis in the delimitation of the clean and proper body, a process that constitutes an awareness of corporeality and bodily boundaries. This awareness centers on the child's acquisition of language, for it is when the child learns the language associated with proper sociality that subjectivity is possible. Through expulsion and exclusion of the improper, the unclean, and the disorderly elements of corporeality, the child can take up a symbolic position as a social and speaking subject. For Kristeva, the processes of subjectivity are "intertextual practices; . . . subjectivity is enacted by way of language" (1990, 175, cited in Reineke 1997, 19).[19]

Although abjection is predicated on the polarizations of inside/outside and subject/object, it is not reducible to these oppositions. What is excluded from the body can never be fully obliterated but hovers at the borders of existence. "We may call it a border," Kristeva writes, but "abjection is above all ambiguity. Because, while releasing a hold, it does not radically cut off the subject from what threatens it—on the contrary, abjection acknowledges it to be in perpetual danger. But also, abjection itself is a compromise of judgement and affect, of condemnation and yearning, of signs and drives" (1982, 9–10). Abjection, as Grosz writes, "cannot be readily classified, for it is necessarily ambiguous, undecidably inside and outside (like the skin of milk), dead and alive (like the corpse), autonomous and engulfing (like infection and pollution)" (1989, 74). It is not either one thing or another (as structuralism would have it), but it is both these states. Abjection, therefore, is fundamentally "what disturbs identity, system, order, . . . does not respect borders, positions, rules, . . . the in-between, the ambiguous, the composite" (Kristeva 1982, 4).

The three broad categories of abjection that Kristeva identified—food and thus bodily incorporation; waste; and the signs of sexual difference—are all located in the existential immediacy of bodily experience. These three key areas are central to the remainder of this book, in that they provide the theoretical tools to examine the ethnographic data.

In the first category of abjection, reactions to it are visceral, for it is via the emotions and bodily sensations of desire and disgust—retching, vomiting, shame, weeping, and sweating—that this concept exists. Of eating and drinking, Kristeva observes:

> Food loathing is perhaps the most elementary and most archaic form of abjection. When the eyes see or the lips touch that skin on the surface of the milk—harmless, thin as a sheet of cigarette paper, pitiful as a nail paring—I experience a gagging sensation and, still farther down, spasms in the stomach, the belly; and all the organs shrivel up the body, provoke tears and bile, increase heartbeat, cause forehead and hands to perspire. Along with sight-clouding dizziness, *nausea* makes me balk at that milk cream, separates me from my mother and father who proffer it. "I" want none of that element, sign of their desire; "I" do not want to

> listen, "I" do not assimilate it, "I" expel it. But since the food is not an "other" for "me," who am only in their desire, I expel *myself*, I spit myself out, I abject *myself* within the same motion through which "I" claim to establish *myself*. That detail, perhaps an insignificant one, but one that they ferret out, emphasize, evaluate, that trifle turns me inside out, guts sprawling; it is thus that *they* see that "I" am in the process of becoming an other at the expense of my own death. (1982, 2–3, emphasis in original)

Unlike Douglas's writings, Kristeva's abjection is located not only on the margins of bodies, but also in the visceral and pulsating movements of her body.

During my fieldwork I found that people with a diagnosis of anorexia had embodied reactions to certain foods remarkably similar to those described by Kristeva. Some shuddered at the very thought of eating; they drew their bodies inward and closed their lips, put their hands over their noses and mouths, closed their eyes, and often said they felt nauseous at the very mention of certain foods. By drawing inward—closing and protecting—participants were evoking disgust and revulsion, an emotive casting out of abject horror.[20] At the same time, many felt the searing pull of hunger, of being engulfed by desire, as Jane described: "Sometimes I think 'I'm not anorexic, I'm just not hungry.' But I am—I'm always hungry. I'm hungry all the time, and I'm so scared that if I give in to my hunger I will never stop eating, that I'll just keeping eating and eating and eating and never be satisfied."

The second category of abjection, the embodied reaction to waste, is also horror toward that which transgresses borders and boundaries and merges with the self. "What goes out of the body," according to Kristeva, "out of its pores and openings, points to the infinitude of the body proper and gives rise to abjection" (1982, 108). Grosz, paraphrasing Kristeva, states:

> Bodily fluids, wastes, refuse—feces, spit, blood, sperm, etc.—are examples of corporeal byproducts provoking horror at the subject's mortality. The subject is unable to accept that its body is a material organism, one that feeds off other organisms and, in its turn, sustains them. . . . For example, feces signifies an opposition between the clean and unclean which continually draws on the opposition between the body's interior and exterior. As internal, it is the condition of bodily existence and of its capacities for regeneration; but as expelled and externalized, it signals the unclean, the filthy. Each subject is implicated in waste, for it is not external to the subject; it is the subject. It cannot be completely externalized. (1989, 75)

Arising from the horror of corporeal waste is the third category of abjection, the signs of sexual difference. Like Douglas, Kristeva argues that not all bodily wastes have polluting value. Tears, for example, although they belong to the borders of the body, are not dirty. Menstrual blood, however, does signify horror, for it "stands for the danger issuing from within the identity (social or sexual); it threatens the relationship between the sexes within a social aggregate and, through internalization, the identity of each sex in the face of sexual difference." Menstruation not only signifies sexual difference between men and women, but also marks the differences between men and the maternal (1982, 71).

Constituting Abjection Ethnographically

While Kristeva argues that she approaches and surveys the concept of abjection phenomenologically, her writing of this concept remains firmly embedded in texts and the language of psychoanalytic theory (1982, 31). As Reineke observes: "The abject typifies the unconscious"; it is uncovered "at the point of cleavage between the Imaginary and the Symbolic" (1997, 22, 21). To illustrate this space, Kristeva draws on mythic, poetic, religious, and avante-garde representations in literature and art to evoke the sensations of abjection. "Outside of the sacred" Kristeva writes, "the abject is written. . . . Great modern literature unfolds over the terrain [of the abject]: Dostoyevsky, Lautréamont, Proust, Artaud, Kafka, [and above all] Celine" (1982, 17–18). Like Douglas's, her concept of sacred draws explicitly on the texts of the Old Testament. Biblical abominations (both semiotic and spoken through confession) construct "the logic that sets up the symbolic order" (ibid, 110).

In many ways, the illustrations that Kristeva gives for abjection demonstrate the limited usefulness of psychoanalysis for this book. As a genre that deals with problematic terms such as "precultural," "ahistorical," and "preoedipal," psychoanalysis, I believe, cannot be constituted ethnographically. To assume such a universalist psychological ordering is untenable, and Kristeva (similarly to Douglas) has been widely criticized for making unfounded generalizations (Butler 1990, 1993; Grosz 1990; Reineke 1997; Spivak 1981; and Tsing 1993).

I do not use Kristeva's psychoanalytic framework.[21] I remain, however, drawn to her concept of abjection, for it has striking resonances with my fieldwork. Experiences of anorexia, like abjection, are fundamentally embodied, ambiguous, and transformative. While these terms—"embodiment," "ambiguity," and "transformation"—are themselves not abject, they are rendered abject in anorexia. Anorexia, as we have seen, plays with and makes ambiguous the relationships of self and other, both through self-identification and in wider relationships. Experiences of anorexia pivot on ambiguous relationships with food, bodily (and other) wastes, and sexual difference. Participants experienced the simultaneous pull of desire and disgust, as well as the horror associated with foods and bodily fluids as they transgressed boundaries. Although clearly not one and the same, anorexia and abjection both "demonstrate the impossibility of clear-cut borders, lines of demarcation, divisions between the clean and the unclean, the proper and the improper, order and disgust" (Grosz 1990, 89).

In the remainder of this book, I extend Kristeva's concept of abjection by constituting it ethnographically through the everyday practices of anorexia. Abjection played a central role in people's experiences of anorexia. This role was not deployed simply through language, but practiced through gendered bodies; the simultaneous hungering for and spitting out of foods; the physical retching of vomiting and purging; the erasure of sexual difference; the protection of bodies from contamination; elaborate cleansing routines (both internally and on the margins of bodies); and the desire to be clean, empty, and pure.[22]

Moreover, this ethnography demonstrates that abjection is fundamentally concerned with relatedness. If, as Kristeva outlines, abjection is concerned with that which is desired and expelled, then it is equally concerned with relations of connection and disconnection. What is desired or expelled (for example, food, wastes, spaces, memories, and people) stands in relationship to the self. This self is not a unified, stable self, but one that is in process and recognizes the dynamic relations of self and other on a number of levels. These are relationships that participants had with their selves (with an otherness within the subject), with other people, with anorexia, and with objects in their worlds. Abjection is thus not solely about individual identity, but also concerned with intersubjectivity, "the ways in which selfhood emerges and is negotiated in a field of interpersonal relations, as a mode of being in the world" (Jackson 1998, 28).

Before extending abjection ethnographically here, I offer some caveats. The first is to distance this research from the potentially misleading reproduction of the child-mother (and in this case daughter) relationship that has been well examined in the literature on anorexia. Some early feminist analyses of anorexia have drawn on Klein's object relations theory, pointing to the mother-daughter bond as instrumental in the development of eating disorders (see, for example, Chernin 1986; Orbach 1986). While several participants did discuss their relationships with their mothers in terms of their development of anorexia (some mothers had eating disorders themselves), these were not the only relationships they singled out. Some also pointed to fathers, brothers, sisters, and aunts as significant in providing familial and familiar contexts for eating-disorder practice. Moreover, as I argue throughout this book, relatedness is not confined to relationships within the family, and my use of abjection does not fall back on the maternal matrix that Kristeva outlines. Rather it is concerned with the broad-ranging possibilities, conflicts, and experiences that any number of relationships provide.

Second, my use of the word "practice" is distinct from Kristeva's; she, as Oliver notes, suggests that "poetic language is text as practice" (Kristeva 1984, 181, cited in Oliver 1993, 3). My use of the term "practice," which is informed by Bourdieu's habitus, focuses on the everyday practices of ordinary living. As Ortner suggests, practice is, for Bourdieu, concerned with the "routines that people enact [and reproduce and transform] . . . in working, eating, sleeping, and relaxing, as well as the little scenarios of etiquette they play out again and again in social interaction" (Ortner 1984, 154). It is thus through the enactment of everyday temporospatial and gendered practices that abjection is found.

The first of the ethnographic contexts for abjection comprises the remainder of this chapter. In moving Kristeva's location of abjection beyond the symbolic, imaginary, psyche, and language, I demonstrate how the anticipation of particular foods generated abjection, that is, the specific qualities of calories, fats, and oils and their embodied responses. While it is essential to outline the properties of foods that people treated as abject (for example, those that continually moved between the categories of solid and liquid), it is equally important to explore how these foods moved in and out of the body and the responses to this movement. It is the interplay of senses that is central to this embodied abjection, for it is through "the medley of senses bleeding into each other's zone of operation" that we come to experience the world (Taussig 1993, 57).

"Are you a fats or calorie girl?"

Like Douglas and Kristeva, I was interested in the nature of dirty and clean foods. Why in Beth's food list was red pepper clean? The answer lay not in the linguistic or structural classifications of types of food, but in the properties of the foods themselves and their embodied effects. Capsicum was clean for Beth for several reasons. First, she had "read somewhere" that pepper contains "negative calories, . . . as in the amount of energy you need to digest it is more than the food itself gives you." And second, red and green peppers were clean because their surfaces and textures were not slimy and greasy. Capsicums were "squeaky clean." In contrast were foods that glistened (such as melted cheese on top of a pizza), or those that left remnants of oil behind. Beth suggested, for example, that if she had to eat foods high in fat she would much rather eat avocado than fried chips, as the nature of greasiness was different. Seeping, greasy foods were considered dangerous, fatty, and dirty.

It was thus the indeterminacy, the ambiguity, of foods that was at stake. Food continually transforms itself through the varied processes of digestion; when heated or cooled; when mixed with other foods; and when left to rot.

Food, as Lupton similarly notes, is "therefore a source of great ambivalence: it forever threatens contamination and bodily impurity, but is necessary for survival and is the source of great pleasure and contentment" (1996, 3).

Interestingly, it was the practices of food avoidance that marked differences and established alliances between people with anorexia. We have seen the relationships that people with anorexia develop with each other, and as an example of the "special language that people with eating disorders share," Tamara explained that when people meet in a treatment setting one of the first questions they might ask each other is, " 'Are you a fats or a calorie girl?' You're usually concerned about both, but one more so than the other, and if you share the same fear of fats there are immediate likenesses. Calorie girls are worried about airborne contagion, whereas the fats and oil girls are concerned with touch."

Participants described fats and calories as contagious because they had the ability to move and transgress boundaries. They had the potential to engulf, contaminate, and merge. Kristeva notes that while all food is liable to defile, it "becomes abject only if it [crosses] a border between two distinct entities or territories" (1982, 75). The concern with contagion was related to the intertwining aspects of abjection—the threat and incorporation of harmful substances, the ambiguous form of particular foods, and the potential for that which is indeterminable to transform.

Miasmatic Calories

The fear of airborne contagion was related primarily to some participants' belief that calories have the ability to diffuse out of food and into the air. Calories were attributed an insidious nature because of their perceived smallness, invisibility, and potential to move. In a chapter entitled "The Forgetting and Remembering of the Air," Abram reminds us of the simultaneous pervasiveness and invisibility of air:

> On the one hand, the air is the most pervasive presence I can name, enveloping, embracing and caressing me both inside and out, moving in ripples along my skin, flowing between my fingers, swirling around my arms and thighs, rolling in eddies along the roof of my mouth, slipping ceaselessly through throat and trachea to fill the lungs, to feed my blood, my heart, my self. I cannot act, cannot speak, cannot think a single thought without the participation of this fluid element. I am immersed in its depths as surely as fish are immersed in the sea. Yet the air, on the other hand, is the most outrageous absence known to this body. For it is utterly invisible. (1997, 225)

While Abram (in a Heideggerian tradition) "illuminates" that which is hidden in the everyday, these two features of air—its pervasiveness and simultaneous invisibility—were paramount in several people's fear of air.[23]

A number of participants told me about a young Australian woman named Bronte who exemplified this fear of "flying calories." Bronte's "struggle with severe anorexia" had been closely followed in the press (both television and newspapers) over several years in the late 1990s. A popular Australian women's magazine, which ran "exclusive" updates on Bronte, quoted some of the "worst times" of her "nightmare": "One thing I remember is that when I first came in here [for treatment] I couldn't walk past anyone who was eating because . . . I felt the calories had gone into me somehow. I'd roll up towels and push them under my door so the calories from outside couldn't come through and go into my body" (*New Idea* 1998, 15).

For Bronte and others with similar fears the most threatening entry point for calories was via the sense of smell. Smelling meant inhaling an essence of food that carried calories. What was even more distressing was that smells moved and knew no boundaries. They circulated through the air, hung in kitchens, or traveled through the house (under doors and through open windows), permeating the rooms. Rita recounted her fear of smelling food in her family home: "Very early in the piece when I smelt cooking in the house—I would have been about fifteen, a teenager—I used to wonder, I used to hope against hope, that those molecules of food smells getting into your nose and into your body didn't actually carry any substance, like calories. I was terrified that it may be fattening to actually smell food—like almost the smell of food is in and of itself intrusive, not just the physical plunging of stuff in; . . . it's another hole that it gets in."

"Did you ever protect yourself?" I asked.

"Yeah—or I left the vicinity," Rita said.

"Did you ever walk into the kitchen and cover your face?"

"I don't remember," said Rita.

"Or hold your breath in the kitchen?"

"Yes," she said, "yes."

As participants' fears of flying calories affected relationships within their families and households, strategies of aversion and avoidance became paramount. Tamara, for example, who enjoyed cooking and preparing meals for other people (with ingredients with which she felt safe), couldn't go near the kitchen when someone else was cooking: "If mum was cooking whenever I was home, I couldn't be in the kitchen. . . . I felt like if I even went near it I was going to catch calories; . . . too many calories flying around here."

Howes's phenomenology of smell explores why the characteristics of this sense are ideally suited to expressing contagion and danger. He argues that smells are distinguished by their "formlessness, indefinability and lack of clear articulation" (Gell 1977, 27, cited in Howes 1991, 140). As a consequence, smells "are always 'out of place,' forever emerging from things [and merging with things], that is, crossing boundaries" (Howes, ibid.). René Devisch, in his ethnography of emotions among the Yaka of Zaire, similarly points to the liminality of smell, "since it evokes and crosses boundaries between different realms of experience. This primal sensory or emotive experience instigates transitions between persons and categories. Smell may evoke strong moods or provoke emotional changes in the individual. . . . Bad smell from decay or smell that mixes bodily functions can no longer mediate between persons, but evokes repugnance" (1990, 119–120).

The fear of food smells might explain their absence in my fieldwork sites. Although fieldwork sites can be saturated with smells (see also Howes 1991; Seremetakis 1994; Stoller 1997), the spaces I encountered in the field were noticeably devoid of such aromas. Only once in someone's home did I enter to the warm smell of biscuits baking in the oven. Vicki, who said that she could only bake now that she was "recovering," was making a batch of biscuits for her father, who was about to go on his annual Easter fishing holiday. More commonly, I found that the only smells in participants' homes were those of antiseptic cleaning fluids, swabbed over surfaces to sanitize and erase odors.

This fear of airborne contagion has resonance with the miasma theory of disease common throughout the Middle Ages and up to the emergence of the scientific model of medicine (Lupton 1994, 33; Corbin 1996). The large number of epidemics and plagues during this time led to an understanding of the body as permeable and highly susceptible to invasion and attack by disease. Disease was likely to be most prevalent where the noxious vapors of miasma were present; for example, the foul, stagnating smells from marshes, bogs, or sewerage works were considered dangerous and believed to cause disease if inhaled. The most dangerous vapors were related to the heat of decomposition, to rotting vegetables, animal, or human waste, where decomposition created "putrid emanations" and "harmful effluvia" (P. Wood 1997, 28). It was when substances were transforming into waste that they were seen as most dirty, dangerous, and potentially harmful.[24]

Miasma, like Kristeva's proliferating corpses, signifies "the utmost of abjection . . . because [it] represents 'a border that has encroached upon everything': an outside that irrupts into the inside, eroding the parameters of life" (Ellman 1990, 181–182). Miasma represents disintegrating boundaries and in-betweenness, threatening to contaminate by connecting separate entities.

"The Snake That Slithers": The Ambiguity of Fats

If for participants the concern with calories is related to their invisibility and invasion through smell, the concern with fats is related to their visibility, their slimy, greasy feel, and their ability to seep and sneak into the body through a variety of means. Fats are, to borrow Douglas's terminology, "the snake that slithers." Like snakes, they have a mode of locomotion that enables them to cross the boundaries of their habitat and move out of their proper place. And like the airborne contagion of calories, fats could move and infiltrate. Participants felt that fats were more threatening than calories, however, because once in the body they would stick and solidify "like cement." Recall the earlier ethnographic example in which Estelle explained how she could eat sugar but not fat: "Sugar disappears, it can be burnt off, whereas fat does not dissolve, it sticks and stays with the body, it can be seen. You think of this stuff here (pinches her stomach) and you think of that as fat, not sugar. . . . I could almost imagine it just going straight onto my thighs, or my bum, or my tummy whereas the sugar I imagine diluting through my system."

Estelle is highlighting the properties—the ambiguous texture and form—which mark fat as polluting. Fat is indeterminate in form, it is difficult to get rid of, it seeps, infiltrates, and congeals. It is liminal in the sense that it can be either solid or fluid; it is in between. Fat is like the skin on the milk that Kristeva described; it is revolting "because it forms the boundary between two elements and two different forms: liquid and solid" (Vice 1997, 165). It connects.

Fat has the power to effect embodied visceral responses. The smell, sight, and tactility of oil evoke not only disgust, repugnance, and nausea for Estelle, but also death. The embodied sensations of fats and oils transport Estelle, as the poet Baudelaire (1975, 42) might say, "back to the event with which it is originally associated," back to the fish-and-chip shop in which she worked:

> I can remember that smell very vividly. It's a foul smell and we emptied out the deep fryers into buckets out the back, and the next day I came back and it was like this layer of fat sealed over the top—solid fat—oooh, that's gross [shakes her head and screws up her mouth]. And it smelt gross. I can remember a pig getting cut up after it had been shot [on the farm] and just that sort of smell—I don't know. The smell of fat burning—it's hard to describe. . . . There's something dead, . . . I don't know. When I think about it, it makes me feel sick—just the smell and the look of it. You can imagine it—the way it settled on top of the bucket—I can imagine it settling on the top of my stomach and it never getting out. Just the way it coagulates like that. . . . It would just stay in you forever and ever and never get out. When you get that layer of grease and you can feel it on your teeth and the inside of your mouth—uugghh. Some girls reckon they can feel it in their stomachs and stuff—I never had that—I can never really feel the food in my stomach, but I can feel the fat and the residue in my mouth or on my lips and it's really greasy.

In Estelle's body, she imagined, fat coagulated like the fat in the bucket. It was matter out of place: "Fat was very much like something under the skin that I didn't want there—like sort of something invading my body and getting in the way of what good muscle could be there. It was just something that shouldn't be there [laughs]—an alien sort of presence."

The clogging effect of fat has resonance with current concepts of health. Before her diagnosis of anorexia Karen had been visiting a naturopath who had prescribed a number of tablets to "cleanse her digestive system." Part of the cleansing routine involved a very detailed attention to food consumption, with cleaning foods such as vegetables and tofu encouraged. The naturopath had advised Karen that eating these foods would cleanse her liver, arteries, and digestive system, which were clogged with fats and hence sluggish. The naturopath told her that she should not have fatty deposits in her liver, and fat in the bloodstream was dangerous because it could be the precursor to a heart attack or stroke. Fats were characterized as "out of place" (by both Karen and the naturopath), potentially dangerous to the flow of blood and bodily fluids, and hence dirty.

Protection from Transformation

The measures participants put in place to protect themselves from the polluting nature of fats were far more extensive than those associated with smell. Protection from smell meant covering the nose or mouth, whereas protection from fats required an elaborate surveillance of the entire body. Because of their seeping and sticking nature, fats were regarded as more insidious than calories—they could enter through any part of the skin, cling under fingernails, or be transferred unwittingly from hand or object to mouth. "They're so slimy and pervasive," recounted Angela, "like they can just sneak into places where they shouldn't be and you just feel that you would never get it out of you. It was going to sit there like a lump spreading its grease all through your body."

One fifteen-year-old, Elisa, who was undergoing a bed program in a psychiatric unit at a major public hospital told me in hushed whispers from her hospital bed that she did something "really weird"—so unusual, Elise said, that she hadn't told the psychiatrists for fear of what they would make of her: "I'd prepare food for my brother and sister all the time and towards the end, like just before I came in here, the last four weeks or so I'd wear gloves or wrap my hands in Glad Wrap [plastic cling wrap] because I couldn't stand the thought of fat seeping into me. [Laughs]. It just seems so silly."[25]

Elise's concern with the amorphous nature of fat tempered the very relationship she had with both food and her family. In the hospital, where she was expected to eat all meals presented to her, she would first check the oiliness of a food by touching it with her fingers (like a piece of blotting paper soaking up a fluid). Elise knew, for example, that a piece of cake would contain butter, but she didn't know how much. She would touch it to feel how much residue it left on her fingers in order to gauge the fat content. This initial assessment of food by touch was far more important to her than the information brought her by her sense of smell or sight, for the amount of oil was the mitigating factor in her response. What Elise called "obvious fat"—the butter in small plastic containers or margarine spread on bread—did not have to be gauged in this way. She once apologized for scraping the butter off her sandwiches and onto the side of her plate as we sat together eating lunch in the patient dining room and explained: "I know this looks pretty irrational and silly, but it's a must."

Elise hated the oily feel of butter—"It's oily, it's greasy," she said, as she made a rolling gesture with her fingers, reproducing the slippery sensation. "It's a dirty feeling. I hate the feeling of when my hands are greasy because you feel so dirty." Avoiding contact with greasy and oily substances was not limited to foods but extended to a range of other objects. She was so concerned about oily substances being absorbed through her skin and congealing in her body that she stopped using hand creams, wouldn't wash her hair with shampoo or use lip balm to moisten her lips. Her rationale at the time was: "Well, where does it go? It disappears into your body and then what?" A media story about Bronte similarly highlighted the fear of greasy cosmetics: "[The nurses recalled how Bronte] wouldn't even allow us to put moisturizing cream on her hands because she thought the oil might have some nutritional quality and would be absorbed into her skin" (*New Idea* 1998, 16). Skin was no longer the first line of defense.

Tanya's avoidance of fats was remarkably similar to Elise's. Instead of wearing gloves when handling food, Tanya immediately afterward washed her hands with soap and water: "If I'm making a sandwich for my brother and sister, I don't even like to get butter on my fingers. I can't even touch it. It's like there's a really irrational piece of me that says, 'You'd better not get it on your fingers just in case it's possible that'—this is going to sound really stupid—'but just in case it's possible that the fat could somehow seep in through your skin.' Even saying it out aloud is embarrassing because logically I know that it is so far from the truth, but you can't stop yourself thinking things like that and it's weird."[26]

Avoiding fats proved to be a difficult challenge for those who worked in the food/catering industry.[27] Tamara waitressed in a pub that prided itself on serving German-style foods (thick steaks and rich sauces) in smorgasbords and counter meals. Initially she said that her repulsion for the fatty foods was due to their high calorie count, but she later admitted that it was also because she was frightened that these substances would "somehow seep through [her] skin." Working behind the closed doors of the kitchen, Tamara would "never go without" the recommended disposable gloves when handling food and resorted to wearing them even when it was not required. "I wouldn't even pick up a bottle of oil or a tub of margarine. I couldn't go near it, the fear was just immense. It was like if I picked it up it would somehow get onto me and into me. It was just this incredible fear that it was going to get me." Like Elise, Tamara reiterated how illogical her fear was, but the imperative to avoid touching fats overrode the irrationality. Rozin, Millman, and Nemeroff (1986), who tested Frazer's and Mauss's laws of sympathetic magic in contemporary settings, suggest that the laws of magic operate even though people know better. The power of metonym and metaphor transcends the dictates of logic and reason.

Another young woman remembers being absolutely vigilant around anyone who was eating in her house. At the dining room table, Vicki refused to let her father pass anything across to her if he had touched butter with his hands, for fear of it transferring to her: "I would flip, I would lose it, if dad touched butter and then went to touch a glass or something I was using. I would make him wash it." To prevent the spread of contamination, Vicki had her own crockery: a specific bowl, spoon, glass, and cup that only she would wash and use.

Other participants were fearful that clean foods would become contaminated by dirty foods through close association on plates or mixed in recipes. At the family dining table, Catherine would separate all the food on her plate, as she believed that greasy foods (such as mashed potatoes) would contaminate clean foods (such as zucchini and tomatoes). She still separates what she eats "into little parcels—so the flavors and parts of the food don't mix." She remembers: "My mum used to think it was weird—everything wasn't allowed to touch each other on the plate. You'd have your vegetables there and something there—the different kinds of foods couldn't touch—all separate and all in their little portions." When I asked her reason for separating the foods, she explained: "I liked to have them separate—this word pops into my head—and so it wouldn't contaminate the other food [laughs]. I still do that today; . . . if I had something on my plate which I didn't like or that was very fatty, it couldn't touch the other vegetables because of the fat might get onto them, you know, so the flavor or whatever was in that food would spread to the other things. Things like the butter and the meat—the meat could never touch the vegetables—agghh."

The food that Catherine had the most trouble with was mashed potatoes. Potatoes on their own were clean, but if milk or butter was added to make mashed potatoes then it was contaminated. It transformed from a "good food" to a "bad food," from edible to poison: "I used to use the contamination thing on the plate [laughs and looks away] or in cooking things. You can contaminate things when you cook things, . . . like adding things in. . . . Eating [the mashed potatoes] I used to think, I'm going to die. . . . And I know I had a few arguments with my mum and she'd make mashed potato and put butter in there and I'd crack up at her, 'You've destroyed it, you've contaminated it—I'm not going to eat it.' "

Fear of Transformation

Fear of transformation was not located solely within the realm of greasy foods. Participants experienced as problematic other foods that had the potential to move and be abject. Becky, for example, was terrified of the color of some foods. Howes suggests that "a color always remains the prisoner of an enclosing form," yet several participants clearly demonstrated that this was not always the case (1991, 140). Becky was the first to explain this fear to me:

> When I was anorexic, I believed that if I ate something red it would contaminate my entire insides. For example, if I drank red punch, I had some fear that it would dye my insides red—my stomach, intestines, liver, et cetera. And because I associated red with dirty, then my insides would be dirty too. Do you see the connection? However, it goes one step further. There were some red things that I could eat: tomatoes, catsup, and strawberries. Those red things don't dye things. For example, if you drop a red jellybean in some water, the jellybean will run and cause the water to turn red, right? But if you drop a tomato in the water, it doesn't run or cause the water to turn red. The things I could not eat were the ones that would run and thus dye my insides. Does that make sense to you?

Why the color red?[28] There are two ambiguous characteristics of red that intertwine. The first is the symbolism of the color, and the second is the ability of the color to move. Becky associated the color red with the fluidity and danger of blood. It was the in-betweenness—the potential for multiple meanings—that invested it with ambiguous properties. "Red is the worst color to me. In my anorexia, I could not eat anything that was red. Red is a contaminant. Red is dirty. Red is all consuming."

Red was also dangerous because of its capacity to move and transform. Dyeing involves a merger of properties and an overlapping of domains. The process fundamentally changes the nature of that with which it merges. The color that Becky ingests, she believes, seeps out into her body and transforms her. She in turn becomes that which she equates with red: dirt, danger, and pollution.

Becoming Like Another

The transformative properties of food, their ability to move and merge with the body through sensory perception and experience, are strikingly similar to Frazer's (1959) and Mauss's (1902) descriptions of magical belief systems. According to Frazer, there are two laws of sympathetic magic: the law of similarity and the law of contact or contagion. Contagion, he suggests, rests on the principle that "things which have once been in contact continue ever afterwards to act on each other" (1959, 7). In magical practices, contagion occurs through a variety of means: direct contact with the contaminated source, indirect contact with bodily products (such as hair, fingernail parings, or spittle), or through touching an intermediary object. Influence of contagion has the potential to be permanent (hence, "once in contact, always in contact") (Rozin, Millman, and Nemeroff 1986, 703).

Frazer's laws of magic describe embodied states of transformation. The whole purpose of magic is of course to effect a change in the condition of the person on whom it is practised (Howes 1991, 130). This change is effected through the senses. The connection between the senses and transformation has been well documented, especially in the case of magic. In the Trobriand Islands, "the sense of smell is the most important factor in the laying of [love or sorcery] spells on people; magic, in order to achieve its greatest potency, must enter through the nose" (Malinowski 1929, 449, cited in Howes 1991, 130).

It was sensory connection and transformation that evoked fear among participants: fear of touch, of drawing in another's breath, or of looking at others. Danielle wouldn't follow in what she called "a fat person's" footsteps for fear of becoming like that person, becoming obese. Like the game that children play avoiding the cracks on the pavement, Danielle could not step on the shadows of others lest she "absorb" their "fatness." Breathing in another's odor also had the potential to transform her into that person. As an example, Danielle described how she doesn't like to stand next to someone who may have a cold or smells of garlic, as she feels by breathing in their smells she will be contaminated. She will either turn away so as not to "share air" with them or take shallow breaths. Similarly, when she travels on a bus and she wants to shut her eyes, she ensures that no one else is in her line of vision before she closes them, as if by shutting her eyes she might incorporate some of their presence.

Mimesis, as Taussig writes in his elaboration of Frazer's laws of magic, involves a playing with, or blurring of, different kinds of bodily boundaries: "One becomes something else, or becomes Other" (1993, 36). Bettina was constantly worried about becoming other. Again, it was through the senses that these transformations were most likely. When eating, she tried not to think of other people, for she feared that the food would take on their properties, which in turn would transform her. She could not stand too close to people for fear of merging with them. For many years she had to eat "flawless" food: "Everything has to be perfect—especially with food. For example, this morning I had a piece of bread with a crease in it. I was unsure of whether to eat it or not, but there was no other bread, so I ate it. Then I became worried if I should have eaten it or not; . . . sometimes I don't know what normal is. Sometimes I can't decide who I am, or where I start or finish. I'm worried that people or objects can influence me, that I can turn into them. . . . I just want to become perfect again . . . and that's how the food is involved—I know that you are what you eat, and that's why what I eat has to be perfect."

As an ethnographic reworking of Kristeva's concept of abjection, in this chapter I have explored the relationships that people with anorexia had with particular foods. Extending beyond descriptions that rely on taken-for-granted discourses of nutrition or mind/body control, the analysis has highlighted a different level of understanding about food. For many participants, food was experienced as abject: as a dirty, disgusting substance that they equated with bodily waste. It was however, not simply the oral ingestion of food that was threatening to participants, but also the possibility of connecting with dirt and contagion through other sensory modes such as touching and smelling.

It was thus foods that had the potential to move and transgress that were most problematic. Oils and fats, for example, were defiling because they moved between categories of solid and liquid. They were the most threatening of all foods, for they had the ability to transgress bodily boundaries through touch, seeping through the skin into participants' bodies and sticking and clogging "like mud." Smelling foods was similarly problematic, for air was a carrier of food smells, a carrier of calories and of contagion.

Having established abjection as an ethnographic focus, I explore in the next two chapters how that which people with anorexia considered abject was cast out from the body. They center on the erasure of disgust and how people cleansed their bodies of dirty, polluting food through purging. Another level of cleansing was related to the erasure of the female body itself. Women described and experienced their bodies, and in particular their reproductive, digestive, and sexual bodies, in the same ways that they described food, as polluting, dangerous, and dirty. Anorexia was a practice that removed the threat of abjection.

6

"Me and My Disgusting Body"

In sixth grade I used to take days off from eating, to cleanse my system.

—Mayra Hornbacher, *Wasted*

Despite being referred to me while she was an inpatient on an eating-disorder ward, Julia disagreed with her diagnosis of anorexia. "It's not anorexia," she told me, "it's an ambivalence to food." Ambivalence was a recurring theme throughout her narrative and the dominant motif on which her relationships pivoted. Thirty-eight years of age, Julia was the fourth child in what she described as "a really bright, high achieving family; . . . it's very hard coming fourth in line to smart, bright women. I'm not suggesting that I'm stupid, but they put unbelievable expectations on me and at the same time treated me like the baby all the time." Her upbringing was at times like "a civil war; . . . we've all got dreadful tempers and we're all very strong willed and obnoxious but we really do love each other."

As an example of the family volatility, Julia described a typical Sunday family lunch. "They were horrendous," she said as she rolled her eyes and shook her head in exasperation. She hinted at the abuse of alcohol and drugs by other family members, and her disgust at that "kind of behavior." She wanted to distance herself from what she saw as their "complete lack of control," a distancing that she effected by choosing not to share in the commensality of family gatherings. She withdrew into "a safe place," where she did not have to engage or partake in intimate relationships. This space was what she called "anorexia"; her "protest against the status quo, against everything."

In keeping with the family luncheon theme, Julia talked of tablecloths, the white, laundered spread at the center of family dynamics that has food passed over it and spilled on it, arms leaned upon it, drunken laughter and angry dialogue thrown across it. Tablecloths continually transform: during a meal they become dirty, and they are later soaked and bleached to return to their original state. As Visser notes: "a good deal of its prestige rests upon the trouble such a tablecloth entails: it must be washed and pressed every time it is used, and a single stain ruins it" (1992, 156). Julia described the different types of tablecloths—the "everyday and the special occasion"—and it was the special occasion tablecloth that she likened herself to: "I guess [anorexia] is like having a really clean, beautiful, embroidered or cross-cut white tablecloth that you would never use because if you did—even though it's there to be used and it's beautiful and tablecloths always get things spilled on them—something is ruined. It's stained, it's spoiled, it's been ruined. . . . I'm like the tablecloth that's wrapped up in tissue paper in the drawer or wrapped in plastic and kept safely away nice and clean but is never used and never admired. I'm not prepared to go so far as to have things spilt on me and the spilling—the spillage is all the stuff that made me and my family miserable."

Julia's story illustrates a number of continuing and interwoven themes that unfold in this book regarding the relationships between dirt, disgust, and cleanliness. In likening herself to a never-used tablecloth, Julia echoed the concerns of many other participants that food has the potential to defile, to pollute, and stain. Wrapped in tissue paper, tucked safely away in a drawer, Julia avoided not only the spillage of wine and foods, but also the spillage of relationships, in her case the turbulent emotions of family life. Through restricting her food intake, she refused to share the cloth of commensality and attempted to remain pristine and clean like the white embroidered linen.

Julia's metaphorical rendering of anorexia is an example of one of the ways in which people diagnosed with anorexia in my research avoided defilement. Avoiding food (restricting intake) and purging (most commonly vomiting or laxative use or both) were the two main ways in which participants protected and cleansed themselves. These practices were clearly positioned in a number of differing discourses. In the medical field, on the one hand they were viewed as markers of diagnosis and severity of illness, as symptoms of a disorder, as a means to weight loss. Historical and feminist analyses, on the other hand, look beyond the signs and symptoms to the wider meanings of purging, exploring the ascetic experiences of fasting saints and other religious groups. These discourses are quite separate in their endeavors: one looks at the physiological ramifications of food refusal and purging (such as weight loss and electrolyte imbalance), and the other at the ascetic separation of the mind from the body in an attempt to reach purity and salvation.

I explore the connections between and beyond these two discourses. When participants talked about purging and restricting, they rarely spoke solely about weight loss or spiritual salvation. Their discourse consistently returned to a desire to be clean, pure, and empty. Restricting and purging cleansed their bodies of that which disgusted them: dirty and polluting food. The logic seems straightforward: food that comes into contact with the body has the potential to become part of the body—to be absorbed—and must be removed. To touch it, smell it, taste it, or eat it is to embody dirt and disgust.

There, were however, other levels of embodied disgust that had to be cleansed from the body: experiences that related directly to gendered bodies.

Bodies and food are inseparable, as I have argued throughout this book, and in the case of anorexia it is the experiences of the female body and food that are inseparable. Women described their bodies, and in particular their medically fragmented bodies—reproductive, digestive, and sexual—in the same ways that they described food: as abject. Although participants described the potential for desires, hungers, and pleasures, they overwhelmingly experienced their bodies as dirty, polluting, and dangerous. Female participants came to feel this disgust through unwanted sexual experiences, by their own bodily processes (menstruation, digestion), and via fear of sexuality. Participants not only wanted to rid their bodies of defiling food, but in the process to erase and cleanse their own "dirty and disgusting" bodies.

Explaining Purging

In the early months of fieldwork preparation, while speaking to clinical directors and health professionals, I often encountered blank faces when I asked about the meanings of bodily fluids. The ways in which people purge—self-induced vomiting, laxative and diuretic use—were viewed as straightforward, self-evident measures for losing weight. As one psychiatrist was signing an ethics approval for my project, he replied in answer to my question: "That's simple, they do it to lose weight." The American Psychiatric Association's 1987 *DSM-III-R* classification echoes his understanding, describing these practices as "abuse so as to achieve weight loss and maintain a low body weight."[1] These practices are thus rendered instrumentally as the signs and symptoms of anorexia nervosa.

Signs of Disease

Signs and symptoms are the bread and butter of diagnosis in medicine. Hippocratic medicine emphasized the careful observation and registration of every symptom, forming the basis for establishing precise histories of each disease, even if that disease was itself unknown at the time (Honkasalo 1991, 251). With the appearance of medicine as the natural science of the body in the eighteenth century, symptoms lost their central place in diagnostic practices, for through them one could only *infer* the disease causally. Symptoms came to be seen as subjective evidence or assessment of a disease, such as a complaint or pain. A sign, by contrast, was seen as objective evidence of the disease, observed, interpreted, and tested independently by the physician rather than the patient.

Foucault refers to this shift in medicine as a "syntactical reorganization of disease" that treats signs and symptoms differently and expects them to cohere into a rationale explanation: "The symptoms allow the invariable form of the disease—set back somewhat, visible and invisible—to *show through*. The sign announces: the prognostic sign, what will happen; the anamnestic sign, what has happened; the diagnostic sign, what is now taking place" (1973, 90, emphasis in original).

Purging is a symptom that has observable and detectable signs to a clinically trained eye; it can be deduced from enlarged submandibular and parotid glands or measured by a number of specific laboratory tests (routine blood chemistry studies or nonroutine assessments such as serum amylase levels) (American Psychiatric Association 2000, 13). As a symptom, vomiting or diuresis allows the clinician to observe the physical signs of malnutrition, to listen to abnormal bowel sounds, or measure a low body temperature.

Purging is an important diagnostic marker, as it also allows further classification into specific types of anorexia. The *DSM-IV* outlines two subtypes of anorexia nervosa: restricting and binge/purging (American Psychiatric Association 1994). Someone who restricts their food and fluid intake but does not take laxatives or diuretics and does not vomit would be classified as having the restricting subtype of anorexia nervosa. Members of this group are known as the pure anorexics among inpatients (see chapter 4). To use Julia's metaphor, they are the special occasion tablecloths, who revere purity. There is recognition in the medical field that anorexics may swing between purging and restricting: "Patients with anorexia can alternate between bulimic and restricting subtypes at different periods of their illness. Among the binge-eating/purging subtype of patients with anorexia nervosa, further distinctions can be made between those who both binge and purge and those who purge but do not objectively binge" (American Psychiatric Association 2000, 19).

From ward rounds and participants, I learned of the telltale signs of anorexia that called one's bluff or gave the game away. Beth and I would sit on the back veranda of her shared house in the late summer mornings, drinking glasses of water and adding cigarette butts to the already overflowing ashtray. She was a pale, thin woman in her late twenties and often dressed in dark-colored t-shirts, baggy pants, and black sandals. At times her voice was faint, and she often looked contemplatively out onto the sparse, dry garden, collecting her thoughts and delivering them in serious and measured responses. During our conversations Beth would always tuck her long legs under her body and place her hands in her lap, playing with them as we talked, picking at her fingers and nails. In her moments of contemplation, my attention was drawn to her hands, and the small sores that were concentrated over the knuckles of the first two fingers on both hands. My first thought was that these marks might be cigarette burns, as several other women had shown me scars on their legs and hands from self-inflicted razor blade and glass cuts. I later discovered that these were "Russell's sign," a medical term for skin lesions consisting of abrasions, small lacerations, and calluses on the joints of the hands (Daluiski, Rahbar, and Meals 1997). These nondescript lesions are caused by repeated contact of teeth and the skin of the hand as it enters the mouth during self-induced vomiting (Zerbe 1993, cited in Hornbacher 1999, 61).[2] When I asked Beth about these marks, she said that the observable signs of anorexia—her lacerated knuckles along with obvious weight loss—were not indicative of her experiences: "They are only medical signs. It's not what it's really about." When I moved away from the domain of semiology mediated by the medical gaze and its language, I began to learn about the ways in which purging was experienced as a polysemous and often contradictory practice. Purging was a means to lose weight, but more significantly it was a means to rid the body of defiling food and erase feelings of disgust. Beyond the taken-for-granted understandings of purging, it was a transformative process that temporarily eviscerated emotional states (of disgust, shame, and guilt) and senses of embodiment (of emptiness and purity).

When I asked participants about purging practices, I received a mixed response. Some rolled their eyes, looked away in embarrassment, or asked me why on earth I was asking. Self-induced vomiting, Nadia said, was not "like throwing up." It was intentional and hidden, and many participants believed it did not signal an illness. "I'm so ashamed of what happened through all those years," Nadia said. "It's not like vomiting normally—sorry, tape [apologizes to my tape recorder]. . . . I think it is such a private thing. I wouldn't divulge everything anyway, simply because it's too hard for me to verbally admit, but you do some amazing things."

"But what's normal throwing up?" I asked her.

"When your body makes you do it," she said. "Most of the food's digested and it's bile and it really smells, whereas I think throwing up after having eaten a lot—and I was really regimented and had to throw whatever I ate up before two hours, before you knew it was going to be digested in four, so I had strict guidelines to follow—and it's not digested and half the time it's not even masticated properly, so it still looks like what it went down as, so it's really different. . . . I used to throw up till I bled, so I was always going to get it all out regardless."

"Yeah, I was going to say, How do you know when to stop or when it's all come out?" I asked.

"Well, you have to drink a lot of water or milk—you have to do it during, otherwise it's just too hard. But when you can taste bile, that's generally a good sign, or when you bleed and there is just nothing else coming out until the water runs clear that you have just drank. It's quite disgusting really."

Many commented on their ability to vomit and purge without others (at home, school, or work) ever being aware. Ellen started vomiting when she was twelve years old, and for the next six years no one knew about her "terrible, dirty secret." In lunch hour at school she would vomit in the toilets: "I got very good at it and I got very quick. I didn't need my fingers after a time and it was just like secondhand, almost, I wouldn't even think about it." Amanda told me how she could easily hide her purging practices from her parents, proudly elevating her techniques of vomiting to an "art form. You do it very quietly—silently, in fact, so no one can hear you." She described the movement of undigested food up through her body: "I can start it just by bending over and just squeezing—you know, if you see a belly dancer squeezing their muscles, it's kind of like that. You start down there and then squeeze gradually up the esophagus, kind of like peristalsis in reverse." To disguise the fact that she was vomiting, she would often turn the sink tap or shower on in the bathroom to fill the silence.

Other participants had never talked about the details of purging with anyone and welcomed the opportunity to speak about such experiences, and a few who had talked about it with therapists and psychiatrists were willing to share their techniques with me. Emily told me how she learned to lavage her own stomach with a length of green garden hose after having her stomach pumped in an emergency department for a drug overdose. "I thought, If they can do it, so can I." She carried around a twelve-inch piece of hose in her handbag so she could lavage at any time.[3] I found it hard to imagine this demure and well-dressed woman with her precision-applied makeup slipping a garden hose down her throat. These contradictory images and the openness of her detailed descriptions surprised me, as I wrote in my field notes at the time: "I was somewhat taken aback by her frank descriptions of the garden hose that she uses to flush her stomach out—in fact she said that she had done this on her way to meet with me (she has the hose in her handbag). She knew all too well the potentially fatal dangers of this practice, she has already perforated her esophagus and had it surgically repaired. She said that it must sound really weird to me, and that doing it disgusts her, but that she is driven to do it as she must get the food out of her body."

Emily had been lavaging her stomach every day for the seventeen years, each time drinking up to a liter of warm water and sometimes adding a squirt of Fairy Liquid washing detergent to help the food "slide" out more easily. Rather than use oil as a lubricant, Emily chose a detergent that doubled as a cleaning agent. I asked her why she felt driven to lavage her body. "It means that I become smaller," she said, "and then there's less of you to contaminate the atmosphere. I feel that I pollute society." When I asked why she felt that, she said: "I have very strong feelings of no self-worth; that is the nucleus of my problems. Sometimes when I eat, I feel the food absorbs the badness and when I get rid of the food I am getting rid of the badness."

Emily liked to feel empty; it made her feel "clean and calm." Feeling clean, empty, and calm were often noted as the immediate benefits of purging, as

Hornbacher remembers of her first purging experience: "And so it came to pass one day, stuffed full of Fritos, I took a little trip downstairs to the bathroom. No one gave me the idea. It just seemed obvious that if you put it in, you could take it out. When I returned everything was different. Everything was calm, and I felt very clean. Everything was in order. Everything was as it should be. I had a secret. It was a guilty secret, certainly. But it was my secret. I had something to hold on to. It was company. It kept me calm. It filled me up and it emptied me out" (1999, 41–42). "Emptiness," MacSween suggests, "means being clean, . . . not contaminated by external things, . . . pure" (1993, 248).

Purging Histories

"Calmness," "cleanliness," and "purity" were terms to which participants returned in our conversations about purging. In describing the need to keep her body pure, Tamara made a direct link between anorexia and the asceticism of medieval Europe. Things that came into the body, she said, like food—"the forbidden fruit"—or sex, carried impurities and would sully a body's purity. She traced this belief through history: "There was the whole monastic era where the monks denied themselves things because they wanted to purge their bodies of everything and be pure and so they wouldn't eat and do this and that, and I think we still have a lot of that in our culture that is sort of unconscious, or comes along those lines of need to keep purity in our bodies, so putting things in that make us either fat or unhealthy is sinful—because that's what they all thought."

These parallels between asceticism and contemporary self-starving practices of anorexia have been vigorously debated in the historical, anthropological, and feminist literature (and to a much lesser extent in the medical literature).[4] "Asceticism" is a term derived from *askese*, "a Greek concept originally developed from athletic training, and modified by the ascetical school of the Cynics and Stoics to mean the practice of conquering one's vices and faults, the control of impulses and self-conquest in preparation for the realization of the moral life" (Peters 1995, 55). It implies a spiritual or religious foundation that relates to self-discipline and resistance to the temptation of food, as exemplified in prolonged fasting (Vandereycken and van Deth 1994, 2).

A number of authors have explored whether contemporary anorexia has links with medieval ascetic fasting practices. The central question is, "Were the medieval fasting saints holy anorexics?" The answers have tended to fall into two camps: those who argue for historical continuity between the practices (Banks 1992; Bell 1985; and Bordo 1988) and those like Bynum 1987, Brumberg 1988, Vandereycken and van Deth 1994, and Lester 1995 who insist there is none (Garrett 1998, 113).

The practices of self-starvation, binge eating, and self-induced vomiting have a lengthy history (see Nasser 1993). Bordo traces the cultural preconditions of fasting and feasting back to the times and writings of Plato, Augustine, and Descartes and the laying down of a dualistic conception of mind and body. She argues that this long heritage constitutes "the basic body imagery of the anorexic" in which they gain self-identification through control of the body: "intellectual independence from the lure of its illusions, to become impervious to its distractions, and most importantly, to kill off its desires and hungers" (1988, 92, 93). Eckermann describes bingeing and vomiting as central features of the wealthier classes in Ancient Rome, where it was considered au fait to visit the vomitorium for group vomiting after feasting. Even earlier, Hippocrates recommended the use of laxatives, emetics, and restrictive diets to maintain the balance of the four humors. The ancient Egyptians purged by way of cow's milk and infusions of fennel, honey, and sea salt for both the treatment and prevention of illness (1994, 83).

Rudolph Bell 1985, Bynum 1987, and Brumberg 1988 trace practices of self-starvation and purging back to the thirteenth century, when food abstinence occurred in close relationship to Christian religion and could give rise to either devout veneration or suspicion of possession. Fasting saints such as Catherine of Sienna were often accused of being witches in league with the devil and supposedly fed by demons at night. To ward off persecution, St. Catherine took pains to eat something during daylight hours to avert accusations of possession (Vandereckyen and van Deth 1994, 35). Similarly, the fifteenth-century saint Columbia of Rieti supposed that she had been possessed. Her vomiting was said to relieve her of evil spirits, "just as she had seen in pictorial representations of exorcisms" (ibid.). Unlike Bordo, Bynum sees "the body" acting in new ways at particular historical moments and argues that there are major differences between the motivations of the holy anorexics and of contemporary self-starvers. Medieval asceticism was not rooted in dualism, and thus an attempt to escape from the body, but was rather "an effort to plumb and to realize all the possibilities of the flesh" (1987, 294).

Yet these writers overlook a fundamental difference between fasting practice and anorexia. One is concerned with a path to connect with the afterlife, and the other is concerned with disconnection from life itself. Religious practices of fasting and food avoidance are related to a very particular *communion* with an afterlife. Iossifides' fieldwork in a Greek Orthodox convent demonstrates this connection. She describes how the nuns in the convent were on "a spiritual journey which they hoped and prayed would lead them to permanent unity with the divine after their death" (1992, 82). To achieve this they renounced major aspects of ties that served to incorporate people within a secular society: ties associated with the body, and kinship ties of marriage and childbearing. Partaking in the ritual of Holy Sacrament (a liturgy and communal meal) united the nuns with Christ and the laity, and "all are members of a blessed community" (85). Relatedness was thus negated on one level (in the everyday world) in order to establish an infinite connection of spiritual relatedness.

Those few participants who did cite religious doctrines as a parallel framework for understanding the purging and restricted eating of anorexia did so, not in relation to communion with an afterlife, but as a disconnection from dirt and life itself. Sonya, for example, spoke of her denial of food in a very particular way: "I feel like I need to deny myself. I need to deny myself clothes. I need to deny myself nurturing stuff. I was raised very orthodox Catholic, where you deny yourself stuff in order to be clean and pure." Purity here is couched not only in a religious framework but also in a moral hygienic discourse. Carolyn, in describing her intense preoccupation with cleaning her body, cited Rev. John Wesley's statement that cleanliness was a virtue "next to godliness" (see also Hoy 1995, 3; Thomas 1994).

Garrett (1998) argues that spiritual/religious backgrounds are central to people's development of (and recovery from) anorexia. Most participants, however, did not use a religious framework to describe anorexia, even those who were actively engaged in church or spiritual pursuits. My concern was not with forcing this connection (a critique that has been leveled at Garrett), but rather with focusing on the language and bodily sensations participants were using to describe restricting and purging, the *purity* and *cleanliness* that being *empty* effected. In not taking a singular religious view, my approach to asceticism is not dissimilar from O'Connor's suggestion that "ghosts of dead religious beliefs" (for example, the Protestant work ethic) live on in "life styles and occupational cultures that reproduce themselves" in a reinvented secular asceticism (2000, 7). I found that participants related purging and restricting practices to dirtiness and disgust—the dirtiness and disgust of food and most particularly of their own bodies. Their desires for cleanliness were not obviously related to spiritual connection and cohesion but were concerned with removing, casting out, and separating from that which disgusted them. Secular asceticism thus recognizes a religious history, and the transformations of this legacy in nondenominational, everyday practices.

Embodying Disgust

In *The Woman in the Body*, Martin suggests that women's imaginings of themselves and their bodies have been shaped by the language and models of medical discourse. This shaping has provided popular perceptions of women's bodily experiences (and most particularly reproductive-related processes such as menstruation, childbirth, and menopause) that are overwhelming negative. Scientific models, she argues, denigrate women's bodily experiences by "implying failed production, waste, decay, and breakdown. Menstruation, for example, is described in standard texts for medical students as a negative process, exemplified by words such as "failure," "deprivation, " "constriction," "diminished," "disintegration," "hemorrhage," "debris," "loss," and "necrosis" (1987, 197, 45).

Participants with anorexia often drew on similar negative metaphors to explain their experiences, describing themselves as like "toilets," "full of shit," "garbage," "scum," and "rubbish." They felt their bodies, like food, to be "out of place," "dirty and polluted," "dangerous," "disgusting," "diseased," "contaminated," "soiled," and "impregnated with evil." More than Martin's metaphors of "failed production," these women experienced their bodies as inherently abject.

The women in this project wanted to cut the flesh off their bodies and be left with the clean, hard "truth" of bones. For Sonya, "flesh" was feminized and associated with excess, sin, and guilt. She wanted to strip away the flesh that she believed had led to her sexual abuse: "Bone is strong and carries no female flesh or semblance of femininity. No man would ever want me." Kristeva similarly notes that "the brimming flesh of sin belongs, of course, to both sexes; but its root and basic representation is nothing other than feminine temptation" (1982, 126). The power of sin lies within female flesh.

In contrast, the men in this project wanted more definition of their muscles. Despite their small numbers, the ways in which men and women spoke about and experienced their bodies was, as one would expect, different. The men did not experience their bodies or bodily fluids as dirty.[5] They did, however, describe aspects of their sexuality as dirty and disgusting, such as a desire to view pornographic materials, masturbation, a fear of being homosexual, and for one young man, the experience of sexual abuse. All three men in this project spoke of their desires and fears around homosexuality, a category that is in itself feminized, marginalized, and in some contexts culturally constructed as "dirty and polluting."[6] This view was fueled considerably by the advent of AIDS and the demonization of contaminating homosexual practices.

The limited data on men's bodily experiences precludes their full inclusion in this argument. What is interesting, however, is the ambiguous positioning of both the men and women in this project (through differing aspects of gender and sexuality). Both were symbolically polluted and polluting. Emily and Estelle, for example, made a distinction (which was not always clear-cut) between the food that polluted their bodies and their selves, which polluted society. Such a positioning for all the women led to a desire to feel empty and clean.

There were various ways in which women came to experience their bodies as dirty and disgusting. Specific events such as unwanted sexual experiences left some feeling disgusted and ashamed of themselves. To be violated was to be transformed into "damaged or spoiled goods," where the only solution was, as Sonya explained in relation to her experiences of abuse, "to be clean and transcend above this hideous society that you can't stand because it's so mean and cruel." Others described their own sexuality and bodily processes (such as menstruation and pregnancy) as disgusting, dirty, and dangerous. Catherine, for example, knew that there was something dangerous about her teenage years, as her parents allowed her brothers to socialize but she was no longer allowed to go out. In justifying their need to protect her, Catherine sensed that her teenage body had the capacity for desire and danger. Beth described anything to do with sex or bodily functions as "unclean." Having periods was "messy," and she remembers her utter disgust at waking up one morning to find that she had "leaked" blood all over her pajamas. She felt dirty after having sex with her boyfriend. Others who felt alienated from families or friends came to feel out of place, worthless, and uncared for: "When you feel like you're not worth anything, you feel like you are the scum of the earth, a real dirtbag" (see chapter 4).

Turning on Disgust

What these experiences have in common is the feeling of disgust. In his early writings on disgust, Rozin claimed that this emotion circulated around ideas of contamination and contagion, a fear of oral incorporation, and food rejection. In tracking this body of work, Miller notes that Rozin positioned taste as "the core sense, the mouth the core location, ingestion and rejection via spitting or vomiting the core actions" (1997, 6). Certainly this is the case in anorexia, the desire for food and the desire to get rid of it. Later, Rozin broadened these core ideas of disgust to incorporate not only food, but also "bodily products and animals and their wastes, and then five additional domains: sex, hygiene, death, violations of the body envelope, and sociomoral violations" (ibid.).

These domains are very similar to that which Kristeva defines as abject: food and thus bodily incorporation, bodily waste, signs of sexual difference, and death/the corpse. All of these involve embodied and visceral responses to disgust that "seem to erupt immediately, spontaneously from the gut" (Probyn 2000, 133). It is precisely because disgust is so visceral that it needs to be distanced, pushed away, or eliminated. Disgust, as Miller notes, "differs from other emotions by having a unique aversive style. . . . [It] constantly invokes the *sensory* experience of what it feels like to be put in danger by the disgusting, of what it feels like to be too close to it, to have to smell it, see it, or touch it" (W. Miller 1997, 9). In disgust we gag and turn away, we cover our mouths, purse our lips, and fend off with our hands. Even our stomachs turn. Things that are disgusting are out of place, too close, dirty, and dangerous.

Disgust is the core sensation on which abjection turns. When disgust comes too close, as in being raped or imbibing dirty food, the body is violated and needs to be distanced. Distancing means reducing it, disconnecting experiences, cleaning it, and numbing it. For Ellen, whose tiny stature always seemed to be further dwarfed by the chairs she sat in, it meant disappearing: "Like I wanted to disappear, honestly. I really felt very ashamed about who I was and I didn't want to be me. I had some bad experiences as a child—I was abused quite a bit and I always thought it was my fault and I thought that I had brought it on and so that meant that there was something drastically wrong with my person, so I just wanted to erase everything that was me—become an empty slate."

The most powerful expressions of disgust accompanied participants' accounts of experiences of sexual abuse. Words were spat out, bodies recoiled, voices trailed off, and anger rose. Some asked me to change the subject or preferred not to discuss the topic at all: "Let's not go there. Can we steer away from that?" At times Natalia became increasingly silent and rolled into a ball; these were the times she could not open her body to speak of the disgust that she felt.

Interiorizing Abjection

The literature that has examined the relationship between sexual abuse and eating disorders suggests that approximately 40 to 50 percent of the adult women who have a clinical presentation report a history of unwanted sexual experiences (Waller, Halek, and Crisp 1993, 873). Despite these strong links, other studies cast doubts over such assertions. Some suggest a much lower prevalence rate (Lacey 1990), and others highlight the high rates of sexual abuse in the general population and argue that any links are simply coincidental (Finn et al. 1986; Gordon 2000; Pope and Hudson 1992).[7]

In light of these criticisms, some studies have narrowed their focus and examined the specificities of each eating disorder, looking at prevalence rates *and* specific diagnostic categories. One such study found a strong association between reported unwanted sexual experiences of one hundred women with anorexia and vomiting/laxative abuse (Waller, Halek, and Crisp 1993). Although cautious in its claims, and reminding readers of the "multi-causal nature of eating disorders," this study has direct relevance to my explorations of anorexia and purging, dirt, and rituals of purification. The researchers ask for further research "to elaborate on the 'links of meaning' between reported sexual abuse and specific psychopathologies of anorexia and bulimia nervosa," such as the nature of the abuse (ibid., 878).

In attempting to avoid assumptions surrounding anorexia, I specifically did not ask participants with anorexia about histories of sexual abuse. Despite this, one quarter of the group spontaneously recounted experiences of sexual abuse to me (including one male participant).[8] Some told me when we first met, and others skirted around the issue, as it was a painful memory to recount. In all the accounts, abuse was viewed as central to their experiences of anorexia. As I mentioned, there came a time when Natalia felt it was important to tell me about childhood abuse if I was to understand "her anorexia." It was what linked all the contexts together. It would explain, she said, the bitter self-loathing and disgust that she had toward her own body.

Estelle's evocative and powerful narrative demonstrates the complexities surrounding not eating. It is not only about sexual abuse, for it encapsulates a number of major recurring themes: rape, sexuality, menstruation, and poor self-esteem—all factors that coalesced to form an embodied sense of disgust. Through her story, we can elaborate the contextual links Natalia mentioned.

Estelle stood out from the majority of people with anorexia in my fieldwork for two reasons. First, she had recovered from anorexia, a claim few could make.[9] Not only had she achieved this goal, but she had wanted to recover, again a claim few could make. Second, she stood out because of her flamboyant appearance, as one of the very few who had a distinctive and alternative style of dress. The majority of people with anorexia I encountered were conservative in appearance; they liked to follow current fashion trends. Their distinctiveness was not in what they wore, but through being anorexic.

Most of Estelle's shoulder-length hair was matted into dreadlocks, and the ends were dyed bright pink, some entwined with silver jewelery. Her bangs were pulled back by clips that sparkled in the light, accentuated by the glitter eye shadow dotted around her eyes. She dressed in club gear, wearing two overlapping black Lycra tops (the outer with the animated Japanese character Astro Boy on the front), and a blue hooded unzipped top. She repeated the layering with two skirts, one long, tight-fitting black skirt with purple sandals peeping out underneath, and a shorter red skirt on top.

As I walked across the asphalt car park to her suburban ground-floor flat, I could hear heavy metal music floating out her open front door. It wasn't often that I heard music in participants' homes. Estelle's flat (shared with her "bulimic friend") reminded me of a typical teenage/student place—posters stuck up on the walls, a chair acting as a stool, a couch covered with a blanket, ashtrays sitting precariously on armchair rests, and a TV and stereo. What was distinctive about her living space was the disarray, the music, and the open front door. Many of the homes I encountered were remarkably ordered and clean (itself an interesting observation that I unpack later); there was rarely music playing, and front doors were never open (except in Natalia's case, when she purposely left the door open to invite danger).

One day, sitting on her living room floor, Estelle and I were discussing why certain foods evoke disgust. She began in general terms. "Food is disgusting," she said, then reflected for a moment and moved the discussion to a different focus. "Um . . . (pause) no, it's more me that's disgusting, this is the thing. Food isn't disgusting—it's me, but I can translate it to food. Maybe I thought that the act of eating food was in a way—I've always thought that eating food was pretty gross. The chewing and the stuff in your mouth. I think it's also the thing of having something in your mouth—uuggh—even the thought of that now [shivers and laughs]—it goes back to the rape."[10]

Walking home from school orchestra practice, Estelle was raped. She was thirteen years old.

> Yeah, so it's more me that's disgusting. . . . like because he [the assailant] couldn't enter me down there because I was so petrified—he ended up forcing me to give him a head job and he came in my mouth and so the thought of putting stuff in my mouth is disgusting anyway. Especially if it's anything long and thin like a banana, I can't. I always felt so dirty. I've always associated food with sex—I don't know how but they are one and the same and it just made me feel dirty sometimes after I ate it. It made me feel like I'd been like impregnated by something—like penetrated on the inside by something I didn't want inside me, something I didn't want to be there at all [laughs].

Estelle often highlighted the coterminous relationship between food and sex and recognized the pleasure, desire, and when forced, disgust, that both can arouse: "They can both be pleasurable or you can see them the other way as well. That's why I'm glad I was never actually force fed [with a nasogastric tube] in hospital because that would almost be like the rape. . . . It's something against your will and you can't really do anything about it."[11]

Counihan notes that "food and sex both have associated etiquette about their appropriate times, places, and persons . . . and they can be dangerous when carried out with the wrong person or under the wrong conditions" (1999, 63). To be forced to eat or have sex is desire that is misplaced. Rape (and indeed any form of sexual assault), as Moreno writes of her own assault in the field, "is a vicious, murderous relation" (1995, 247). "A prevalent notion in many societies," Moreno continues, is "that women are themselves to be blamed for rape." This stems from the idea that "it is the responsibility of women to make sure that they are not 'in the wrong place at the wrong time.' In other words, there are times, places and situations out of bounds for women, which they traverse only at their own risk" (219).

Being in the wrong place was exactly how Natalia's experiences were construed by others. In her diaries, Natalia wrote that her mother repeatedly questioned her after Natalia was raped as a child: "What were *you* doing in there? How could *you* let him do that?" Natalia swore to me through gritted teeth: "I will *never* forgive my mother for asking those questions, for blaming me." Women are deemed at risk and often culpable when out of place.

Clinicians frequently pointed out in Estelle's case notes the causal link between her development of anorexia and the rape, an association that Estelle herself was later to come to terms with. For many years after the attack, thinking and talking about certain foods was traumatic for it returned her to that presence, to the touch, taste, and smell of the rape. The thought of sticky and greasy foods still makes her feel nauseous, as it reminds her of holding the stranger's semen in her mouth: "Yuck [laughs]. It's got that dirty, unable to wash it off feeling. It's got the same texture—I don't know if this is going a bit far—but it's got the same texture and look and everything as grease. It's white and gooey, just like fat [laughs]. It [semen] smells and looks disgusting." Grease and semen are interchangeable in Estelle's register of disgust. It is their similitude, their closeness of association, that revolts.

Estelle continued to describe a series of events that compounded and confirmed her own embodied sense of disgust. Following the rape, her grades at school plummeted and she failed her second year of high school. She started to shoplift and take amphetamines, and at fifteen she left the family home and entered a series of abusive relationships:

> I really thought I was disgusting because I had all these people telling me I was disgusting. . . . My first boyfriend would tell me that I was hopeless in bed and he felt disgusted after having sex with me and stuff like this, so I sort of had this real feeling that I was disgusting because that's what everyone kept telling me. . . . The teachers said I was worthless, . . . this Vietnamese boyfriend I had was constantly reinforcing that I was worthless—I was *just a woman*—that somehow something was wrong with me because I was a woman, and then there was the rape, which just made me feel disgusting anyway. So I had all these things telling me I was disgusting. . . . I had my boyfriend beating me up but I felt I couldn't leave him, so I was disgusted in myself for staying with him and being so needy of him . . . and I translated that not so much into my mind being diseased but my body being diseased and I felt like I had to clean my body out. Like I felt that the only way of me not being disgusting would be to sort of not be here in such a physical sense, if you know what I mean. Maybe if guys didn't look at me in a physical sense as a woman then I wouldn't be as disgusting—I'd be an equal to them or whatever. I wouldn't be seen as a slut or as just something to have sex with or beat up and discard, which to me is something you do to a piece of rubbish—which is disgusting. . . . I felt like I had to somehow make myself better because I had all these people telling me how horrible I was, how awful I was, how much of a slut I was or whatever, and I didn't know how to change myself on the inside.

Like Julia, Estelle drew on metaphors to convey her experiences. And like Julia's use of the tablecloth metaphor, Estelle chose one that drew on concepts of dirt and cleanliness. Estelle said that her sense of disgust was akin to a toilet, as her body had become a receptacle for waste. What was put into her (food, sexual organs) and placed on her (criticisms) resulted in her embodying a sense of disgust: "I didn't know how to change myself on the inside so I had to change myself on the outside instead. Cleaning yourself from the inside—somehow like you clean a toilet—flush it. You feel like a toilet or that you're being used like a toilet—being shat on [laughs] and having things placed in you that you don't particularly want there and stuff like that."

The only way to reduce the disgust, which was intimately tied to her sense of womanhood, was to reduce her physical presence and stop putting things into her body. She disconnected from bodily experiences that disgusted her: eating, sex, intimacy, emotions, and the memory of the rape.

Others who have experienced sexual abuse use the same language of disgust and disconnection. In setting the scene for her book, Garrett writes of her own disgust and separation, which began in her childhood.[12] In her introductory chapter, entitled "Personal Sociology," she writes:

> On the aeroplane which brought us back to Australia, I was sexually abused in the cockpit by an acquaintance of my father's; an Australian judge. Heaving with nausea, I pulled my very pregnant stepmother into the cramped aircraft toilet and told her what had just happened. In the sixties, people did not talk about such things. At least she believed me. What he had done was wrong, she said, but some men were just like that; they could not help themselves and there was nothing to be done about it. I would have to put the experience behind me and get on with my new life in Australia. Only my parents knew what had happened and neither of them ever mentioned it again. After a few weeks, the nausea went; but the disgust with my body, the fear of its sexuality and of men were still there two years later when boys began to ask me out. In self-protection, I had separated myself from the source of my troubles—my body—and was frightened by its demands. (Garrett 1998, 8)[13]

Disconnection and alienation from bodies was a recurring topic of conversation with participants. A Canadian art exhibition that visually explored people's experiences of eating disorders had an installation of a dismembered female body entitled *My Body Does Not Belong to Me*. Tamara referred to herself as "me and my disgusting body," suggesting that her body was separate from her self. Participants often used language in this way as a tool for distancing. It allowed them to separate their sense of self from their bodies (rather than saying "I," many referred to their own experiences in the third person). Interestingly, all the men and women in this project referred to their sexual bodies by way of distance—"You know, the bits down there," "nether regions," or "private parts."

When participants disconnected themselves from these types of experiences, they separated not only from the source of their troubles, but also from relationships with other people. Estelle spoke of problems with intimacy and sexual relationships, lack of networks, and loneliness. Ellen, who blamed herself for attracting unwanted sexual attention, distanced herself from all relationships by literally disappearing and hiding: "I just thought that if there was more of me I would command more attention from other people and since I didn't have very good experiences in the past I was worried of what sort of attention of what I might get—or that I might cause someone to do something wrong. . . . I boarded up my windows with black cardboard paper. I never put the lights on and put candles on. . . . I was living a recluse life really."

The Horror Within

Other ways in which women reported feeling that their bodies were dirty related to bodily processes such as digestion and reproduction. At a conference I attended on the history of food and drink, a prominent Adelaide chef commented on the changing obsessions of bodily cleanliness that she saw among her female staff: "People are so scared of dying of cancer or high cholesterol that they go on detox diets. They [the female staff] are cleansing their alimentary canals because they feel their bodies are dirty. In the sixties for me menstrual blood was dirty—now it's people's stomachs and intestines as well that are dirty."

Bodily processes are marketed as a dirty business. During the period of my research, Adelaide's *Sunday Mail* and *Advertiser* both carried a naturopath's advertisement that claimed: "A surprising fact is that few people realize their bowel is the gateway through which dangerous bacteria enter their bodies. Most illnesses, no matter where in the body, start in a contaminated bowel; . . . your quality of life can be dictated by your bowel. It is hard to be the life of the party if your bowel is not performing properly." The advertisement touted a "new bowel cleansing formula that flushes your body of harmful toxins and parasites fast." As well as toxins and parasites, the bowel contains "dangerous bacteria, decaying wastes, poisons, and even meat that is decomposing like a dead body." It is "a sewer, a dustbin, a breeding ground . . . and it causes illness, disease and death." The parasite-attacking herbs and multi-cleansing fibers that are recommended "supercharge your digestive system and rid the bowel of unwanted wastes, toxins, restore bowel health and eliminate parasites" (*Sunday Mail*, February 12, 2000). They work "like an intestinal broom, scrubbing and sweeping the inner walls of your colon" (*Advertiser*, November 28, 2000).

While these advertisements are directed toward both men and women, there is growing evidence that it is women's bodies in particular that are construed as dirty and in need of cleansing. Many participants echoed these fears. A naturopath had told Grace that "her system was blocked" and she "needed to flush it." A plumber would use exactly the same language in regard to a blockage in a domestic toilet system. Grace's meticulous adherence to the recommended diet and her concern with bodily cleanliness were what her general practitioner and psychiatrist blamed for the development of anorexia.[14]

When I asked Amanda how she conceptualized what happened inside her body, she answered without a flicker of hesitation: "My insides are dirty." "Insides" to Amanda were her alimentary canal (her stomach and intestines) and her lungs: "My first thought was of them being dirty, kind of black and dark. I also thought after that of lungs, and obviously they're pretty dirty because I smoke—I thought of that ad [television commercial] where they squeeze the fat and tar out, which I can't even watch—it's obscene."

Several others had no concept of the "journey of digestion" beyond the stomach, as if "a cork was placed at the bottom of [their] stomach." These women believed that food traveled straight from the stomach to their outer flesh, where it stuck fast like cement.

Bettina was horrified at any "goings on" in her body. She watched my pregnant body with fascination, openly apologizing for her own embodied and spoken horror at the very thought of being pregnant herself, an unlikely event, she joked, as "I have an aversion to putting things into my body."[15] She leaned across a table in a crowded coffee shop and whispered to me: "Being pregnant would absolutely—I don't know how I'd cope. Something growing—like growing—it's like, not a fungus, it's a parasite that's feeding off me. . . . It's taking from me and it's sucking me and I feel like it's drawing it all from me, my life is going. . . . It's like in the sci fi movies where something takes over you. It's awful for you to hear me say that."

The thought of something growing, moving, and feeding within me fascinated and simultaneously repulsed her, I was the quintessential abject maternal body. She tentatively asked if I could feel the baby kick and move (quick to point out that she did not want to feel "my stomach"), and when I said I could she put her hand to her mouth in shock, saying it made her feel sick and squeamish. In fact, whenever we talked about bodily processes—secretions, digestive systems, or reproductive systems—she screwed up her face and closed her eyes.[16] She couldn't bear to think of "things moving inside [her]" and wanted to think of herself as completely empty.

A moment later Bettina drew back in her chair and held her arms and hands out in front of her in disgust at her own periods: "I don't like to think that those things are happening, I don't like to think that my body is working inside, in fact, that makes me feel ill; . . . it makes me feel sickly. I'm never sick, like vomit, but it just gives me a feeling of wooziness all the way through, from the pit of my stomach all the way through. Something's happening in there and it's best that I don't focus on it and that's the only way that I can get away with it now is not to focus or think that it's happening."

Although Bettina was horrified at the thought of being pregnant, her home displayed an obvious desire for and fascination with children. Standing in the spare bedroom of her apartment I commented that although she was adamant that she would never have children, much of her house displayed a passion for children's things: the miniature crib made up for a baby, the small tea sets that she had collected since childhood, and her elaborate wall display of dolls (arranged "in order with [her] life"). These objects however, remained at a distance—the crib was in its original plastic wrapper, and all the dolls were out of reach behind glass doors. They were only to look at and not to interact with. Like Natalia's display of Japanese objects, what was important about these objects was their smallness. To take up less space, be "a little fairy," "fit into the size of a matchbox," or to simply disappear was an aspiration. Bettina explained that she loved the dolls because, "like children, they are small, don't speak and have perfect skin and features." Babies were appreciated for their smallness, as Rita said as she touched my pregnant belly: "I love babies because they are so small and perfect."

Coming into New Gender Relations

Bettina's disgust associated with her periods is not a new phenomenon. Much of the ethnographic and feminist literature that explores concepts of menstruation has focused on the constructions of taboo (supernaturally sanctioned law) and pollution (symbolic contamination). Within these frameworks, menstruation is negatively constructed as "the curse" or, more fully "the curse of Eve: a part of God's punishment of women for Eve's role in the Biblical Fall" (Wood 1981, cited in Buckley and Gottleib 1988, 32). Ussher similarly notes the maligning of menstrual blood: "Whether menstruation is deemed to be a woman's relic of Eve—the punishment for the Fall—or merely a biological phenomenon which is inherently debilitating, the taboo ensures that, within patriarchal culture, menstruation is conceived as a curse. . . . Our blood marks us as Other—as we bleed we fail, we fall" (1991, 22).

More recent ethnographic work has criticized the universalizing and reductionistic analyses of menstruation, arguing that "its symbolic voicings and valences are strikingly variable, both cross-culturally and within single cultures" (Buckley and Gottlieb 1988, 3). Symbolic analyses of pollution are limited, for they have obscured the ambiguity and multivalence of women's experiences of menstruation. A framework that focuses on social facts has not only reduced understanding of menstrual blood to a universal biology, but also failed to explore the many and changing social relationships that menstruation brings into play.

While critically appraising the earlier contributions to menstrual symbolism, Buckley and Gottleib (1988) argue that ethnographic specificity is required to redress some of the limitations in previous works. Emily Martin's work perhaps exemplifies this new approach to menstruation. She does not deny the usefulness of past theories or claim a singular alternative; rather her ethnography examines the different ways in which women's reproductive processes are perceived, ranging from dominant scientific ideas to women's own everyday experiences and understandings. For example, Martin describes the positive aspects of menstruation as a "sweet secret; . . . it is clear that women construct the significance of menstruation in terms of the range of opportunities open to them and their expectations about how they will make use of them" (1987, 101–103).

As in Martin's work, I found a variety of understandings of menstruation at play among participants—positive, negative, and ambiguous. The range of responses revealed the range of experience—many women were not menstruating and others had just had their periods return (one after an absence of twenty-eight years). What all the women had in common at one time or another was an absence of periods. Amenorrhea, the cessation of the menstrual cycle, is a major diagnostic criterion of anorexia. "In postmenarcheal females, amenorrhea, i.e., the absence of at least three consecutive menstrual cycles" is a symptom of anorexia nervosa (American Psychiatric Association 2000, 20).[17] Women who think or hope they have anorexia also weigh this diagnostic marker as a defining signal that they have the credentials to join the club. Amanda expressed her delight at "losing her periods": "I lost my period for a fair while, which was good because that meant that I had lost enough weight and maybe I was anorexic."

Having her period signified womanhood, a state that Amanda was trying to avoid: "I think periods signify womanhood, in a way, and I feel like what I'm doing sometimes is getting back to childhood, and that's why I got such pleasure in not getting my period." This explanation concurs with much of the medical literature that suggests anorexia is a fear of sexual maturation and a retreat into childhood. Amenorrhea is said to be symptomatic of this retreat, a rejection of adult femininity (Malson and Ussher 1996, 506), a failure to accept female psychosexual maturity. Such a perspective locates anorexia within the individual, divorced from cultural, historical, and social contexts and relationships.

This was, however, not a common explanation for lack of periods among the women I worked with. Hornbacher strongly argues against the interpretation of regression:

> Too often the shrinks assume an eating disorder is a way of avoiding womanhood, sexuality, responsibility, by arresting your physical growth at a prepubescent state. . . . The shrinks have been paying way too much attention to the end result of eating disorders—that is, they look at you when you've become utterly powerless, delusional, the center of attention, regressed to a passive, infantile state—and they treat you as a passive and infantile creature, thus defeating their own purpose. This end result is not your intention at the outset. Your intention was to become superhuman, skin thick as steel, unflinching in the face of adversity, out of the grasping reach of others. Anorexia develops when a bid for independence on the part of the child has failed. It is not a scramble to get back into the nest. It's a flying leap *out*. (1999, 68, emphasis in original)

The most common understanding among those with anorexia in this study related not to regression into childhood, but to cleanliness. Like many women, participants spoke of periods as "a messy and dirty business" and were glad to be unencumbered by the associated embarrassment and shame of menstruation (Martin 1987, 93). Menstrual blood itself was construed as "not real blood," dirty in comparison to the clean, bright red blood that circulates in the cardiovascular system. And participants often "felt dirty and bloated" when they had their periods. For Rita, menstrual blood, like any form of bleeding, indicated that "something was wrong. The first time it happened, I thought I was dying, it shouldn't be happening." For her, it was blood that was out of place.

The concept of menstrual blood as out of place is at the heart of arguments put forward in works such as Grosz 1994, Martin 1987, Kristeva 1982, Shildrick 1997, and Vertinsky 1994, to name a few. Women, these authors argue, have been aligned not only with a lack or absence, but also with seepage and uncontrollable liquids. "For the girl," Grosz argues, "menstruation, associated as it is with blood, with injury and wound, with a mess that does not dry invisibly, that leaks, uncontrollable, not in sleep, in dreams, but whenever it occurs, indicates the beginning of an out-of control status that she was led to believe ends with childhood" (1994, 205). Tamara hated the way in which menstrual blood "oozed out" over several days and wished that "there was another way it could come out." Her suggestion was to "just get it out all in one go, like going to the toilet and urinating rather than having it drag on." Having it drag on meant days of feeling "a lot worse about myself because feeling bloated and just the bleeding and it's dirty and yuck and inconvenient."[18]

Despite the negative experiences of periods, Tamara simultaneously highlighted the positive aspects of removing polluting wastes from the body: "In a sense it's another act of purging, really, because it's getting out all the gross things; . . . so for me, being a cleanliness freak, I'd rather have it out than in."[19] Estelle similarly described the benefits of losing "dead blood. . . . I sort of used to like it after my period because I felt like I'd lost a bit of weight and lost a bit of blood out of my body. . . . It's been lining the walls of your womb for a month or so and it's dead and it's sort of sticky too. You think it's dirty, so it's good to get rid of it."

Lack of periods was also welcomed because it meant not having to deal with sanitary products. Few participants used tampons, as they "just didn't seem right," were "uncomfortable," and were "not supposed to be there." Beth had only used tampons once. "Never again," she said. "I really doubt that I'd be able to get one in now that I've got this problem with not having enough moisture down there. . . . I think I'd feel really weird with one inside me anyway, walking around with something constantly inside me." The thought of using tampons made Tamara "feel nauseous—like squeamish. I can't bring myself to do it. I think, This isn't right, this isn't natural, and I can't do it." The sense of impregnation or transgression of the body echoed with the descriptions of imbibing foods and was thus avoided.

Related to the onset of periods was a newfound awareness of changing relationships. Houppert suggests that some "people immediately perceive a girl who has begun to menstruate as being different, and girls are treated differently once they've started menstruating" (1999, 109).[20] These changes are concerned with the young girl's coming into womanhood, her capacity to reproduce. When Catherine started to physically develop as a teenager, she sensed a palpable change in household relationships. She had been raised in a strict Baptist family and was taught that sex was "only something that adults did within the sanctioning of marriage." When she started to develop breasts and have periods, she became aware of new possibilities: "Part of it was the family I grew up in. Being a young woman or a woman is dangerous. It's kind of like the feeling you get—boys are out only after one thing and it was too hard, dangerous."

"Why dangerous?" I asked.

"Dangerous because you could get in trouble."

"You mean trouble as in sleeping around or getting pregnant?"

"Yeah, that sort of thing," Catherine said. "It was like it wasn't seen as a good thing."

This idea that menstruation is directly associated with reproduction is part of a wider conceptualization of women's biological grounding. When asked what they understood by the term "femininity," participants designated the arbitrary biology of sexual difference—"the so-called secondary sexual characteristics—the filling out of breasts and hips, the growth of pubic hair, and perhaps most strikingly, the onset of menses" (Grosz 1994, 203). This difference was primarily experienced as negative, as just described, for a body "which leaks, which bleeds, which is at the mercy of hormonal and reproductive functions" is one filled with dread, shame, and embarrassment (204).

In their discourse analysis of interviews with women who had been diagnosed with anorexia, Malson and Ussher reveal that menstruation was negatively construed as a signifier of "femininity" (1996, 509). They argue, however, that it signified a very specific femininity that was alien, out of control, highly emotional, sexual, vulnerable, and dangerous. What is rejected in anorexia is not adulthood or femininity per se, but this particular construction of femininity. My research similarly found this list of constructions at play when women described femininity or womanhood. What this list does not include, though, is the prominent theme of disgust that participants voiced, of bodies that are dirty.

Not all participants had experiences of sexual abuse, abhorrence at the thought of ever being pregnant, or feelings that their sexuality was dangerous. What all participants did experience at some level, however, was disgust with their bodies, and it was the embodiment of disgust that signaled something that was both out of place and too close. Disgust, Probyn writes, reminds us of "the overwhelming horror that the disgusting object will engulf us, [that we have] been too close to things which we prefer not to speak; . . . disgust illuminates the body's capacity for reaching out and spilling across domains that we would like to keep separate, or hidden from view. . . . Basically bodies become too close, to themselves and others. . . . In other words, in disgust, things, categories, people are just too close for comfort" (2000, 131–132).

My fieldwork was redolent with "things which we prefer not to speak." Depending on the context, anorexia itself was recognized as shameful, as something to hide and deny ("I'm fine really, I've just had gastro."). Sexual assault was also not spoken about. Estelle returned to school the day after her rape "to make it look as if I'd just had a sick day, to hide the fact that I'd been raped." Natalia never again spoke with her parents of the assault that occurred while the family was visiting friends. Both distanced the experience, and it was many years before they were able to speak of it.

Disgust was a central element of participants' experiences of anorexia. Disgust points to the abject relations that participants had with food, their own bodies, and other people. In coming too close for comfort, disgust points to the dangers of relatedness.

I have argued here for an alternative rendering of purging that is based on the relationships among disgust, dirt, and cleanliness. Rather than simply a means to lose weight, purging was experienced by participants as a practice that maintained the clean and proper body that Kristeva outlined. Purging eliminated that which "spilled across domains"; it was a movement toward emptiness and purity. The disgust associated with leaking menstrual blood, transgressing sexual taboos, and even chewing and digesting food were distanced and disconnected from bodies.

As Malson and Ussher (1996) argue, these women were removing themselves from a particular discursive construction of femininity. However, in turning the focus away from discourses of individualism (of bodily control and autonomy), these women were rejecting very specific processes of connection. In rejecting the biological grounding of their bodies, participants were rejecting connections of relatedness. Periods, pregnancy, childbirth, and sexual relationships fundamentally connect people. When menstruation ceases, the capacity for childbirth is negated. As one of Eckermann's participants explained: "I have *produced* a body which *denies* sexuality. . . . I have stopped having periods so I can't even have a baby" (Eckermann 1994, 88, my emphasis).

As the cross-cultural literature highlights, it is these processes of sexual maturation that position women in new relationships with others. This positioning was often experienced by participants as disgusting, threatening, and transgressive. Participants did not want to connect with other people. On the contrary, they wanted to be "out of the grasping reach of others." They achieved this disconnection through cleanliness, emptiness, and purity.

7

Be-coming Clean

> The dizzy rapture of starving. The power of needing nothing. By force of will I make myself the impossible sprite who lives on air, on water, on purity.
>
> –Kathryn Harrison, *The Kiss*

Purging through self-induced vomiting and taking laxatives was only one of a range of practices participants cited for cleansing the bodies they experienced as dirty and disgusting. Other techniques included washing and scrubbing parts of one's body with water or antiseptic cleansers, or sucking antibacterial lozenges to cleanse one's "contaminated" mouth. The goal was a body that was sanitized, scrubbed, and exfoliated of experiences, memories, and its own corporeality. These combined washing and flushing practices led me to reexamine the experiences of anorexia under the lens of hygiene.

Bathrooms, toilets, bedrooms, and kitchens were the household sites where these anorexic cleansing practices took place—the sites where bodies and spaces were most intimately related. Despite the great interest in the anthropology of the body, it is only recently that connections between gender and architectural spaces have come into the field's analytic spotlight (see, for example, Butler and Parr 1999; Low and Lawrence-Zuniga, 2003). In their edited collection, Carsten and Hugh-Jones suggest that, like the body, the houses in which people dwell are so commonplace and familiar that ethnographers hardly seem to notice them. They may be part of our initial survey of who lives where and who does what in each space, but they "soon fade into the background to become merely the context and environment for the increasingly abstract and wordy conversation of ethnographic research. . . . In time, for both anthropologists and their hosts, much of what houses are and imply becomes something that goes without saying" (1995, 4).[1]

Inspired by Lévi-Strauss's writings on "house societies," Carsten and Hugh-Jones go beyond the assumed priority of kinship or economic dynamics of houses to focus on the complex ways in which social and cultural relations are manifest in the domestic sphere. This, they argue, enables them to see houses "in the round," focusing on "the links between their architectural, social and symbolic significance." Linked in intimate and conceptual ways, "the body and the house are the loci for dense webs of signification and affect and serve as basic cognitive models used to structure, think and experience the world" (1995, 2, 3).

As I show in this chapter, experiences of anorexia cannot be entirely understood without an analysis of spatial practices. Domestic houses were an idiom of habitus for participants, places where they learned about the pleasures and dangers of cooking and sex and the cultural logic of privacy and hygiene. Bourdieu's concept of habitus extends beyond discursive approaches of hygiene, for it allows an investigation of how people use and transform household spaces and hygiene practices in their everyday lives, the gendered nature of hygiene, and the emotional investments with which cleansing is imbued. The intersecting domains of hygiene—spaces, gender, and emotions—structure this chapter. It becomes clear that hygiene is more than a discourse; it is a taken-for-granted everyday practice that can transform relationships and emotional states.

Comorbidity or the Logic of Practice?

To counter abjection, many women developed highly routinized cleaning practices such as hand washing and teeth brushing. Following a suggestion by her doctor, Bettina meticulously documented the times during the day that she would wash her hands, and what thoughts prompted her to do so. The resultant diaries were recordings of her daily routines in a hospital ward, detailing when she washed her hands, the length of time, and what triggered the washing. All the triggers related to what Bettina considered dirty and contaminating: for example, anything to do with food (she had to wash her hands before and after eating), washing her body (she washed her hands before, during, and after washing her face, before and after she showered, before and during brushing her teeth), when she overheard another patient say a "dirty" word (swearing or slang), when she thought of words such as "fat," "devil," or "pig," and after using cosmetic cream.

The amount of time that Bettina and many others spent cleaning their bodies and houses suggested to me that there was more to this than first appeared. While psychiatric circles saw these behaviors as symptomatic of obsessive compulsive disorder, I began to ask people why they washed themselves (and why particular body parts), in what location they washed, what products they used, and how it made them feel.[2] Rather than view cleaning from the perspective of illness, I took my interpretive cues from participants' themes of purging and protection from disgust and dirt. Cleansing was a way of disconnecting themselves from relationships with other people, memories, experiences, and themselves.

In ward rounds at hospitals, staff made frequent references to obsessive-compulsive behaviors by those with anorexia. The medical literature on eating disorders clearly highlights this phenomenon (Davis et al. 1998; Thornton and Russell 1997; Zubieta et al. 1995), some even regarding "obsessionality and obsessive-compulsive symptoms as important characteristics in the clinical presentation of eating disorders" (Zubieta et al. 1995). While obsessive-compulsive disorders manifest in behaviors, it is thought that these "disturbances" are generated by neurochemical changes, specifically the shifting levels of the chemical serotonin in the brain (Jarry and Vaccarino 1996).

Despite this neurological evidence, I found no exploration in the clinical literature of the connection between anorexic practices and obsessive behaviors. It was taken for granted that the obsessive behaviors associated with anorexia, which were termed "rituals," were part of an associated condition, obsessive-compulsive disorder, often said to have a deleterious effect on treatment outcomes.[3] However, approaching some of these obsessive behaviors from an understanding of abjection (from both food and one's own body), the connections between these practices associated with the separate clinical categories of anorexia and obsessive-compulsive disorder are illuminated. Why, for example, did so many people with anorexia have very particular concerns about contamination, washing, cleaning, and order, rather than the other common obsessive behaviors like checking or counting?

Amanda explained how difficult it was for her to wash her hands after eating because there was no running water in her single hospital room. She would ask the nursing staff for two separate bowls of water (one to wash her hands in after touching food and the other for ablutions), as well as using baby wipes (less effective than washing) to clean her hands of contaminating fats. "I always wash my hands after every meal, or even half way through a meal," she said. "After the main meal and before a dessert I'd wash my hands." Asked why, she replied, "It wasn't the calorie thing, it was just more a dirty thing. I just felt dirty that it had got on my hands, and particularly something like butter."

Rather than categorizing her behavior as an effect of neurochemical fluctuations, I suggest that cultural ideas of cleanliness and hygiene are motivating factors and play a central role in the desire of Amanda and other participants to be empty, pure, and clean. Only once during my fieldwork did I hear these illness characteristics linked. A visiting psychiatrist at a ward round presented "an interesting case" of a young woman who had both "florid obsessive-compulsive disorder and anorexia." What was most interesting about this case, he reported, was that the young woman had fears of food contamination that prevented her from ingesting food and compelled her to repeatedly wash her hands after touching food. The psychiatrist surprised me by remarking that this was an unusual case, for many of the women with anorexia whom I had spent time with had similar fears and responded in a similar way.

It was the combined washing and flushing practices that fascinated me. It was the doing that was important—the washing, flushing, and purging of bodies and spaces that made the transition from dirty to clean. As Kirmayer states: "The meaning of words and gestures is grounded in bodily experience. Meaning resides not exclusively in the relationships between concepts [such as dirtiness or cleanliness] (as structuralism would have it) but in their connection to the body and its skills and practices. Meaning emerges from the capacity to use bodily experience (including socially embodied experience) to think with metaphorically" (1992, 334). Thus the metaphoric relationships among food, dirt, and cleanliness are intimately connected with the ways in which participants experienced their bodies in space and time.

Tamara, at twenty the youngest married participant, was studying full time and lived in a small house with her supportive partner. She described the transition from dirty to clean when she explained her daily "symbolic rituals of purification." She showered twice a day, first washing herself with soap and then exfoliating her skin with a "scrubber." This exfoliation was to make herself "cleaner" and "to take that disgusting feeling away. . . . I'm trying to get rid of the gross, dirty, shameful feeling that's often there." Her partner, Angus, who was fully aware of Tamara's daily struggles with anorexia, gently challenged her on some of these practices. He would remind her, for example, that it was unnecessary to wash her hands in between applying the three facial products she used in her daily "facial routine."

There was a very particular order to Tamara's washing, predicated on what she referred to as the "clean and dirty parts" of her body. She fetched a blue towel from her bedroom to explain the routine to me: "One side of the towel is to dry my face, upper body, and arms [not her breasts or underarms] and the other side is to dry the other areas [she hesitates]—my female parts." She had developed a way of hanging the towel over the towel rail in the bathroom so she knew exactly which side she was using at any given time: "The side with the tag on it is for the clean parts and the other is for the other dirty parts." Tamara also used two washcloths for the same reason. The "dirty parts" of her body—her genitals, breasts, bottom, and underarms—were sources of contagion, pollution, and dirtiness.

For Tamara, the significance of the washing was not only to make her skin appear clean, but also to ease the tremendous guilt, shame, and disgust she felt. Her routinized hygiene practices temporarily alleviated these emotions, which she has had, she said, ever since she was raped by a male friend in her own home. (I return to the emotive qualities of hygiene practices later in this chapter.)

Tamara was using cultural rules of hygiene to wash away her own sense of disgust. These arbitrary principles of hygiene, which are learned in the spaces of the domestic home, are taken for granted and hidden in the persuasions of cultural logic. The dialectical interaction between the body and house is central to Bourdieu's writings, most particularly to his schema of habitus and socially informed bodies. In *Outline of a Theory of Practice* he specifically explores the inhabited spaces of a house, which he terms the "privileged and principal locus for objectification of the generative schemes" (1977, 89). It is in the house that children learn the rules of hygiene—of washing their hands before mealtimes, of bathing and teeth brushing, of cleaning up—and the etiquette associated with the private spaces of hygiene. In analyzing these schemes, or spatial organizations of gender, hierarchy, and division, Bourdieu argues that it is necessary to look at the relationship between the social organization of the household and bodily incorporation if one is to understand the art of living (Warin 2000, 120).

Using Bourdieu's analytical vantage, exploring the spaces most often associated with anorexia reveals them as embodied spaces heavily invested with cultural frameworks of hygiene.

Abject Zones

Staff at the Eating Disorders Association (EDA) had given me some flyers for a play that was to be performed at a small city venue, invited me to attend and also asked me to advertise the event. I attended *What is the Matter with Mary Jane?* on its opening night, sharing a drink with friends and staff from EDA in the small foyer before taking my seat. The performance focused on the life of a young woman who was, the flyer explained, "in the insidious clutch of an eating disorder." The sole performer (her singularity emphasizing the isolation of her predicament) delivered an exhausting one-hour monologue, loudly voicing her embattled desires and fears about her body to the mirror in her bedroom, the audience, and her absent mother and friends.

The stage was demarcated by three domestic spaces: kitchen, bathroom, and bedroom. With no visible walls, these spaces were separated by objects that spoke of the bodily functions of eating, purging, and sleeping. On the left of the stage was a bare, oblong kitchen table, in midstage a white toilet (with a toilet brush next to it and a shower curtain behind it), and on the far right a single bed (with weighing scales that slid under it, a full length mirror, and weights and magazines on the floor). The character, who was never identified by name, moved freely among the three spaces, crying on her bed, vomiting in the toilet, and bingeing in the kitchen on vitamized drinks and food.

Onstage were the three quintessential domestic sites in which anorexia was practiced, and it was in and between these three sites that the eating disorder starred.[4] The absence of architectural boundaries between the performative spaces—no walls, doors, or roof to conceal or contain—was of course necessary for the audience to view the intimate spaces of this young woman's life. We were privy to practices that would normally be hidden from view—vomiting, frenetic bingeing, and hopping on and off scales. Voyeurs sitting in the dark, we watched the constant back and forth movement of her world.

Performing Spaces of Anorexia

As I mapped out the stage in my field notebook, I reflected on the relationship between these staged spaces and my fieldwork. Meanings that had significant resonances with my fieldwork experiences underlay the ways in which the spaces were arranged. It was via the physical opening up of intimate stage spaces, my observing of the movement between spaces, that connections and disjunctures between bodies, places, and practices began to (e)merge.

As in the stage play, bathrooms, bedrooms, and kitchens were key sites in my fieldwork. It was in these three places that bodies were paramount and where practices of secrecy, privacy, sexuality, and hygiene were most overtly performed. Each space was potentially a site of pleasure and desire: the kitchen of eating and tasting, the bedroom of sexual pleasure, and the bathroom a space "for pampering the naked materiality of the body" (Yao 1993, 3). Sibley notes that the pleasures and comforts of home are often given priority in analyses of space. A domestic home is traditionally characterized as a haven, "a place of certainty within doubt, a familiar place in a strange world, a sacred place in a profane world" (Dovey 1985, cited in Sibley 1995, 93). Bachelard's *Poetics of Space* conveys an image of home as comforting and restorative, as a happy memory recalled in dreams, "giving access to the initial shell which shelters the being" (1969, cited in Sibley 1995, 94). Yet while homes can be experienced as cosy, they can also be sites of violence, child abuse, oppression, and depression.[5] More importantly, for this argument, they can be sites of abjection, where tensions confined in spaces change the social relations of those who inhabit them.

In his exploration of the relationships between bodies and space in the Australian home, Yao refers to the bathroom as "a room named desire," a "space that celebrates sensuality and arousal while at the same time encapsulates security and privatization of experience." Rather than straightforward pleasure, for Yao there is a dialectic at play in this space, for the "sensuality of the bathroom is as liberating as it is confining; its aestheticization is concerned with taming the body that is temporarily opened up to arousal" (1993, 3).

A dialectic was at play in the key fieldwork spaces as well, for as each can register pleasure, it can also can register disgust. In participants' homes it was kitchens, bathrooms, and bedrooms (rather than living rooms or hallways) that were most ambiguous and dangerous, for they held contradictory tensions. In each, the body's permeability was heightened, through the ingestion of foods (in kitchens), expulsion of wastes (in toilets/bathrooms), or exchange of bodily fluids (in bedrooms). In each space, bodily boundaries were crossed, transgressed, and transformed. These embodied places were therefore abject zones; they were ambiguous places of transformation, where desire and disgust, pleasure and fear and dirt and purity coalesced.

Moreover, the bathroom and kitchen were spaces of the home that were demarcated as important sites in "the battle to maintain bodily boundaries against contamination. . . . As settings for physical sustenance and hygienic care, the kitchen and the bathroom—and the product 'worlds' they frame—are crucial to intimate bodily experience, helping to form the individual's sense of cleanliness and filth, taste and distaste, pleasure and shame. These rooms are the home's most heavily invested 'objects' of domestic labor: failure to meet the high standards of hygienic maintenance attached to them is a source of guilt and embarrassment" (Lupton and Miller 1992, 504).

Reconfiguring Spaces of Relatedness

These physical and conceptual boundaries between bathrooms, kitchens, and bedrooms, although historically separate rooms (for example, one does not find a toilet located directly off a kitchen), were not distinct in participants' experiences. Spatial boundaries within the home were rearranged; bedrooms became kitchens, and bathrooms became dining rooms. Participants were using spaces that were already signaled as private (bathrooms, toilets, and bedrooms) to purge and hide, and transforming shared social spaces within the home (such as the kitchen) into a private space.

When participants did enter kitchen spaces it was often on their own terms, alone and at a time of their choice. Suzi remembers shutting all the doors to the kitchen in her family home—"so it was all private"—and cooking cakes that she would then take hours to meticulously decorate. If her parents or younger brother came into the kitchen while she was making cakes she would lose her temper and scream at them, for to be disturbed around food, or "caught eating," was a grave invasion of privacy.

Suzi's family became angry with her when she ate alone in the kitchen, so she simply refused to eat with them at all, or even allow them to prepare food for her. Her negating of family mealtimes was an affront to her parents, who were "believers in that saying 'the family that eats together stays together.'"[6] What Suzi was effectively doing was breaking the social bonds that nurturing created within her family (see also B. Turner 1984, 195).

Suzi transformed the intimate space of her bedroom into the single space in which she stored, prepared, ate, and expelled food. "I was buying in tons of food," she said. "My wardrobe was like stuffed with packets and packets of crisps, packets and packets of biscuits, anything sweet—biscuits, cakes, ice creams—my wardrobe was stuffed full. My whole life was spent in my bedroom, to be honest. That's where I lived all the time." As well as hiding food in the cupboards, she spat and vomited into plastic containers that she hid under her bed. Her bedroom was not simply a place for sleeping but also a dining room, a kitchen, a pantry, and a receptacle for bodily wastes.

For participants, part of the retreat to the bedroom was related to the difficulty of sharing domestic spaces, of having to deal with the sociability surrounding food preparation and eating. Elise knew that her mother would "go spare" (be angry) if she found her wearing rubber washing-up gloves while preparing food. It was easier to avoid people by withdrawing to a bedroom. In family homes and shared houses, bedrooms were places that were deemed private and disconnected from others.

Bathrooms and toilets were similarly private spaces, and these were sometimes transformed into eating spaces. Lara discussed the difficulty of sharing a house with another woman, outlining her strategy of taking food to the bathroom. Late at night she would take one apple from her "stash"—the "mountain of apples" in her bedroom—to the privacy of the bathroom, avoiding the commensality of eating. It was a transformation not only of spatial practices, but also of time, for she only ate late at night when the stillness of the house ensured absolute privacy.[7]

Amanda preferred to use the bathroom space for taking lengthy showers not only to cleanse her body, but also to vomit. She would sit crouched on the floor of her en suite shower, vomiting into the drain hole and "poking it" through the grate to be swept away via the plumbing. The water hitting her back from the shower assisted in washing the vomit away, and the sound of it splashing on the floor acted as a cover to the noise of her retching.

A similar playing or remapping of spaces is explored in Angel and Sofia's psychoanalytic treatment of the 1990 film *The Cook, the Thief, His Wife, and Her Lover* directed by Peter Greenaway. The film, which Angel and Sofia describe as having a "voluptuously dirty" aesthetic tension of beauty and violence, produces "an extraordinary mobility and confusion of organs and spaces and the things that go in and out of them" (1996, 475–479). As in the stage performance of *What's the Matter with Mary Jane?* and the domestic rooms just described, there is in the film a connection and disconnection of spaces:

> There is a fluid tracking of the camera from the dark, wet and blue outside, where there are dogs, a naked man, raw meat and fish, in via the scullery, through the predominantly green and yellow kitchen where a multitude of culinary operations are proceeding, and via two smaller red vestibules (from which the [pristine white and overilluminated] toilets are accessed) into the sumptuous red interior of the restaurant,

> past tables laden with artistically arranged delicacies; . . . this arrangement of spaces in the restaurant could be imagined as analogous to the gut, taking in the raw from outside, washing, plucking, chopping, stirring and baking it, then conveying it to the tables where people stuff their faces and afterwards . . . go to the toilet and feed the sewers. (Angel and Sofia 1996, 477)

There is not only fluidity to these spaces, but also blurring of the practices that one would normally associate with each. The kitchen, for example, is not only a site of culinary transformation, but also an important venue for erotic activities: two of the main characters in the film have sex in the kitchen pantries. In a similar vein, the toilets—whose luminosity is reminiscent of the clean interior of a refrigerator or the clinical surfaces of operating theatre (ibid., 478)—are also locations for clandestine sexual encounters. Throughout the film, connections between eating, excrement, and sex are constantly interchanged, collapsed, and placed in direct positions of tension. This tension, Probyn argues, "produces the politics of eating and sex as complex and ambiguous, not to mention downright messy" (2000, 74).[8]

This film plays with key features of abjection. Disgust and desire are continually placed side by side, epitomized in the final scene, in which the main character, who derives great pleasure from eating, is forced to eat a boiled dead body (which happens to be the corpse of his wife's lover) in the dining room. The pleasure of eating is countered by the disgust of eating human flesh. Cannibalism then, is the ultimate abject horror, the pleasure of eating erased by the visceral disgust at eating oneself.

In my fieldwork the tensions associated with abject living spaces were most obvious when participants were confined to their bed in treatment programs. In one psychiatric ward the single side room (of four square meters) conflated all spaces: it was the bedroom, the bathroom/toilet, and the place where patients ate. As such, it was a site that was profoundly ambiguous and confusing, for it was a private side room yet the most public of spaces. I noted this conflation in my field notes at the time:

> There was something "odd" about the space of the single room. On the psychiatric ward of this major public hospital there are 8 beds dedicated to patients with eating disorders. Those who sign contracts with the staff to do bed programs are allocated a single room—a room which contains a bed, a side locker and a cupboard. Nearly all patients transform these rooms into bedrooms—Elise's room, for example, was heavily decorated with posters of Silverchair on the walls and doors, many cards and letters (some from a friend with anorexia whom she had met in hospital and who was also a participant in my research), photographs of school friends, craft pieces, puzzles, a radio cassette

player, a television, candles, gifts from visitors including dried bunches of hanging flowers (arranged in a line above her bed). Her parents had brought in her pillows and duvet from home, adding the final touch of transformation. Like many high-rise buildings, the windows do not open, and the view is of the bricks of the adjacent building. There is a sink, but it has no taps and the plumbing underneath has been removed. This is to ensure that patients cannot vomit or throw food down the sinks. The door to the en suite bathroom is locked for the same reason, and patients are brought bedpans to use on a chair. The door to the room should remain open at all times so if you were to be surreptitiously exercising you would be seen and given a warning and the only time it can be shut or the curtain pulled across is when you need to use a bedpan. Activity is restricted to a minimum and bed rest is encouraged. The single room thus becomes the bedroom, the bathroom/toilet, and the place where people eat—it is a conflation of what is otherwise sharply demarcated in the private and public spaces of suburban homes.

For Beth, the difficulty of living in such a space related not only to the conflation of its functions, but also to the intimate surveillance of her bodily practices and the inability to wash herself:

> The problem with being on the bed in the hospital is that there's no running water—there's nothing—you can't wash whenever you want to, you have no freedom that way. You've only got these stupid, pathetic little baby-wipe things which don't make you feel clean at all so. If they [the staff] were there and they made me spread my jam onto my bread and pick it up and eat it, there was like this jam left on my hands and it was awful because I couldn't get rid of it—even if I wiped my hands it was still sticky—it wouldn't go until it was licked or something. . . . You'd have to dispose of it. It was an extra bit of food that you'd have to try and get rid of because it was there and come hell or high water you didn't want to lick it off, . . . but it might stay there and get into your body.
>
> I have noticed in hospital that there is a bowl of water in the sink. That's for basically washing your hands after you've used the bedpan. I just found that crusty anyway because it's not changed. It's the same bowl of water all day. It's changed every day, but like you go the toilet and you have running water so it's different when you're at home.

"How did you feel about using a bedpan?" I asked Beth.

> I hated it. I hated it with a passion. I hated it. I felt totally awful about it. I thought it was disgusting. I hated using my bedroom as a toilet for

> a start. I also found it quite degrading and disempowering—like they even know when you needed to go to the toilet, they even knew what you did when you went to the toilet. . . . It's just awful. You have visitors and you become really aware of the smell and you're embarrassed. I know a lot of the girls in the hospital are younger but you do get older ones and—not that it makes that much difference but [pauses]—all your independence is taken from you, all of it. You're completely dependent, right down to the "Nurse, I need to go the toilet," you know. That really doesn't make you feel too good. You feel like you're about five. It's awful. I remember once using the bedpan and the nurse coming back in and saying, "You need to drink more. Your wee is very concentrated." And I thought, Oh my God, thank you, thank you—do I have no privacy? It's bad enough that you know when I need to go, but now you're looking at it—it's terrible. I guess it's their job, but it's embarrassing, very embarrassing. But I got through it; I survived it; I live to tell the tale!

The privacy associated with the private single room was a misnomer. Positioned directly opposite the nurses' station, occupants of each side room could be observed around the clock. The surveillance afforded by the architectural design of the ward and the placing of eating-disorder patients in single rooms close to the nurses' station is reminiscent of Foucault's description of Jeremy Bentham's design for the Panopticon (Foucault 1977; see also Eckermann 1997, 157). The resemblance between prisons and inmates, hospitals and patients, has not gone unnoticed, as Bartky, reading from Foucault, writes: "Each inmate is alone, shut off from effective communication with his fellows, but constantly visible from the tower. . . . In the perpetual self-surveillance of the inmate lies the genesis of celebrated 'individualism' and heightened self-consciousness that are hallmarks of modern times" (Bartky 1988, 63).

There are, however, subtle and important differences between Foucault's Panopticon and hospital surveillance.[9] One participant, who at forty-four years of age hated "being treated like a child," crawled on her hands and knees out of her room, along the floor on the other side of the nurses' station, and to the smoking room down the corridor so she could have a cigarette. This creative and resistant act belies the "docile bodies" that are emphasized in Foucault's work. Moreover, in hospitals and treatment centers it was not simply the private lives of patients becoming public, it was a complete reversal of practices: what was deemed private became public, and what would normally be associated with sociality became private. When a patient was eating, for example, as I noted earlier, I was asked by the nursing staff to leave the room to "give them some privacy."

The Threat of Public Spaces

It is no coincidence that the public spaces that posed the most problems were those that participants deemed to be dirty, unhygienic, and dangerous. Public toilets, supermarkets, and hospitals were the main contenders, for objects in these shared spaces had been touched and handled by strangers.

Hospitals, which supposedly epitomized the height of sanitation, were viewed as a "minefield of germs." The thought of having to use crockery, bed linen, towels, toilets, and showers that had been used by others literally terrified people. Amanda considered the hospital to be dirtier than a public toilet: "I won't touch the toilet seat [in a hospital]. If I have to put the toilet seat up or down or whatever, I'll get toilet paper and hold that around it. . . . I hate being in the bathrooms here. I hate them—just because so many people use them and I think that they're filthy. I just imagine all these little bacteria everywhere—uugghh. What concerns me is people's cleanliness, their levels of hygiene. I don't know if they're washing their hands or pissing on the seat. . . . I might catch something."

"And what might that something be?" I asked.

"Nothing definite," Amanda said. "Not like any disease that I know of. I don't know, it's just like catching dirtiness—dirty and contaminating. Not just like in the bathroom but in the kitchen and other places—like if I touch something then I have to wash my hands because otherwise I can almost feel something on my hands, like they feel dirty to me until I've gone and washed them."

"How do they feel?"

"Just like there's kind of a gritty layer on them and you kind of get a bit of increased sensation under your fingertips as if something's got up there and it's dirty."

"And what do you wash your hands with?" I asked.

"Just with Sapoderm soap," Amanda said. "It's antibacterial."

Tamara recounted the high-level negotiations required by public toilets when she stopped at petrol stations on a road trip to Melbourne. She couldn't use the "soggy soap" sitting on handbasins or touch the button on the soap dispenser, so she would always take her own cake of soap in a plastic container. Bettina, when living with her parents and younger brother, had to wash her hands with her own "personal" soap after washing her hands with the soap used by her family.

Carolyn was similarly fearful of the potential for contamination that could be transferred from hand to mouth in public spaces. She was amazed to see other people walking through a food market, choosing a piece of fruit, and eating it. She explained why she washed "every little skerrick [tiny bit] of her fruits and vegetables" before eating them, even the skins: "Even rockmelon and bananas. . . . I wash oranges too. . . . I have to wash the outside; . . . you see, you touch it with your hands. . . . With a banana you can peel it with your hands and the inside might be clean but then your hands may not be clean—it's strange really."

I asked Carolyn why washing foods and cleanliness were important to her, and she immediately spoke of her strict Baptist and conservative middle-class upbringing. As a teenager in the 1950s she and her three siblings were not permitted to wear makeup, dress in the current fashions, eat junk food, listen to popular music, or watch commercial television. Her parents considered these activities to be associated with sin, waywardness, and temptation. What was valued in Carolyn's upbringing was order, restraint, propriety, and cleanliness: "We were brought up with cleanliness—Mum was very particular. Everything was perfectly clean, perfectly. The next-door neighbors used to come and look at Mum's washing and say, 'Beautiful, beautiful' [laughs]. That's why I've got a thing about washing. I just like to be really clean. It makes me feel better." These values have become part of her everyday routines—of her habitus—and she reproduces and practices them without reflection.

At stake in all these spaces—kitchens, public spaces, hospital rooms, and bathrooms—were the embodied cultural practices of hygiene. These practices, however, were constantly under threat from that which was considered abject: foods, wastes, sexual fluids, and people's own bodies. Hands and mouths, as the foregoing examples highlight, were central to the transmission of dirt and subject to rigorous and repeated washing. As Vigarello notes, the focus on the threat of contamination from such body parts has a history: "The bodily zones traditionally the concern of treatises of manners (hands and face, mouth and teeth) were rapidly adopted by treatises of hygiene at the end of the century [1880–1900]. It was on the fingertips, under fingernails or in the grooves of the parts of the skin that touched that microbes were counted" (1988, 205).

The exploration of the changing history of hygiene that follows indicates that the embodiment of taken-for-granted rules of cleanliness played a central role in participants' everyday lives and experiences of anorexia. It was through hygienic practices that they reordered and transformed the threat of abjection.

The Gendered Habitus of Hygiene

Disgust over bodily effluvia and concern with keeping clean through bathing, washing, and antiseptics, pervasive as they are today, have not always held sway. In his beautifully detailed work *Concepts of Cleanliness: Changing Attitudes in France since the Middle Ages*, Vigarello highlights the complex historical intersections that produced contemporary hygienic practices, including differing representations of the body and advances in medicine. A history of cleanliness, he suggests, should first "show how new requirements and constraints gradually emerge. . . . It is a history of the refining of behavior, and of the growth of private space and of self discipline: the care of oneself for one's own sake. . . . On a wider plane, it is the history of the progressive pressure of civilization on the world of direct sensations. A cleanliness defined by regular washing of the body supposes, quite simply, greater sharpness of perception and a stronger self-discipline" (1988, 2).[10]

Vigarello warns, however, that representing this process as "an accumulation of pressures brought to bear on the body risks giving a false picture; . . . such a history needs to connect to other histories, and the most important history in this case is that of the body. . . . Cleanliness is inevitably affected by images of the body"(3).

To highlight the central importance of changing concepts of the body, Vigarello explores the use of water as a cleansing agent. In the Middle Ages in Europe, skin was assumed to be porous, and the prevailing image of the body was one of openness. Water, and particularly hot water, was rarely used to cleanse because "the body had less resistance to poisons after bathing; . . . it was more open to them. It was if the body was permeable; infectious air threatened to flood in from all sides" (9). As a consequence, steam baths and bathhouses were forbidden and water was rarely used to clean the body.[11]

In a time of epidemics, plagues, and the miasma theory of disease, porous bodies needed to be protected. It was clothes, and most particularly their shape and nature, that were all-important in this protection: "smooth fabrics, dense weave and close fit. Infected air should slide over with no possibility of entry" (10). Writing in Paris in 1623, Citoys wrote: "One should wear clothes of satin, taffeta, camlet, tabby and the like, with hardly any pile, and which are so smooth and dense that it is difficult for unwholesome air or any sort of infection to enter or take a hold, especially if one changes frequently" (1623, 20, cited in Vigarello 1988, 10).

Practices of hygiene and, in particular, practices of cleanliness could not be considered without reference to these assumptions (10). In bodies that were swaddled in cloth, cleanliness related to the limited, visible parts of the body—to the face and hands. To be clean was to have no dirt on the surfaces of these external areas of skin. Cleanliness was more a matter of appearance and the social etiquette and "decency" of social relations than of sanitation (46) and was achieved by "dry washing," by rubbing the skin with scented linen. "To cure the goat-like stench of armpits, it is useful to press and rub the skin with a compound of roses," that is, to wipe vigorously, applying perfume, but not actually to wash (17).

Elias (1982) argues that with the internalization of courtly manners (of whiteness and cleanliness), dirt and filth began to arouse feelings of disgust and intense bodily effects (cited in Laermans and Meulders 1999, 119). This was particularly evident among the aristocracy and ascendant middle classes, who shared the symbolic power of fresh, white linen and neat appearance. They considered themselves "civilized," "whereas the popular masses appeared as filthy and thus were to be avoided" (120). Class (and no doubt race) relations were clearly embedded in the value-laden hygiene discourse, where those less fortunate were taught how to maintain standards of cleanliness.

According to Vigarello, these ideas of cleanliness changed in the mid to late eighteenth century with emerging ideas on health, the body, and medicine (see also Thomas 1994). The real transformation that introduced the decisive change derived from the argument of health; cleanliness was a matter no longer of appearance but of health, vigor, strength, austerity, and morality (Vigarello 1988, 228). The body, rather than being perceived as passive and vulnerable to external forces as was the case in the Middle Ages, became endowed with endogenous power and vitality which could easily be released by such activities as cold bathing (128; see also Lupton 1994, 34). Emphasis was upon opening the pores rather than keeping them covered; the goal was to "free the skin" by removing dirt, perspiration, and oils that blocked the surface exits (131–141).

From the 1880s onward, cleanliness was legitimated by the scientific discovery of microbes. Microbes were viewed as "invisible monsters capable of breaking down the body barriers" (204), all the more dangerous because of their invisibility and microscopic smallness. Frequent washing of the body's "nooks and crannies" was needed to remove the dangerous and infinitesimal "bacteria, protozoa and viruses" (202, 207). External signs of cleanliness were no longer considered sufficient (Lupton 1996, 34), and clothes that were not on view, such as underwear, became more important than white collars. Perrot writes in his history of clothes that clean underwear was not only "more hygienic" but also "healthier" (Perrot 1984, cited in Laermans and Meulders 1999, 120).

The hidden danger of pathogenic organisms had profound consequences for social life and social relations. According to Vigarello, "the microbe thus materialized the risk and identified it; . . . the consequences were inevitable: to wash was, as never before, to operate on the invisible" (Vigarello 1988, 203). Regular disinfection came into prominence in public institutions (especially hospitals) and domestic spaces—boiling, steaming, and chemicals were used to clean dirty fabrics, surfaces, and bodies. Private interiors changed to accommodate this newfound attention to body cleanliness; locked bathrooms, washrooms, and bidets became private sanctuaries of hygiene. Taking a bath, it was said, and the resultant washing, constituted one of the best disinfectants. In the terminology itself, washing slipped into asepsis (204). For each of these changes to concepts of cleanliness, an accompanying change occurred in the ways in which people related to each other and to differing spaces.

The core themes that Vigarello discusses in this history of cleanliness saturated my fieldwork. When talking about experiences of anorexia, participants spoke about their bodies, nutrition, and spaces through a lens of hygiene. Their bodies and bodily processes were dirty and disgusting; certain foods were dirty and unclean; private and public spaces (as described in the first section of this chapter) were dangerous sites of contamination. Concepts of dirt and cleanliness embedded in hygienic practices fundamentally changed participants' social relations with themselves and others.

Healthy Homes and Healthy Families

There are a number of aspects of hygiene discourse that Vigarello has overlooked, however, and these are crucial to my approach: the central roles of gender, emotion, and embodied spaces. I turn to gender first. Women and men are involved in hygienic practices in very particular ways (see also Donzelot 1979; Martin 1987, 201; Burke 1996; Laermans and Meulders 1999).[12] While men like Louis Pasteur and Joseph Lister may have had the scientific knowledge to discern bacteria and microbes, it was, as Hoy points out in her history of the pursuit of cleanliness in the United States, the domestic woman who was the agent of cleanliness: "By the 1850's [Americans] were coming to see that cleanliness would be maintained in the family through the agency of the 'true woman' and maintained in the community through public boards staffed by men who were leading citizens in a virtuous republic. Thus, when Americans (urban, [white] middle-class ones, at least) talked about being clean, their conversations generally focused on health, women's work and role, good social values, and the proper goals of public policy" (1995, 7).

Woman's role—that of wives, daughters, and domestic servants—was intimately associated with establishing and maintaining cleanliness. In 1864, during the U.S. Civil War, the *New York Herald* proudly claimed that "all our women are Florence Nightingales" (Hoy 1995, 51). Such a sentiment paid tribute to the role not only of female nurses in the fight against disease and infection at the fronts, but also of the thousands of women who were involved in the work of the Sanitary Commission and *Sanitary Bulletin* back home. The Commission collected and distributed supplies to the front—"soaps, sponges, towels, bandages, sheets, and undershirts," thereby inculcating and maintaining habits of cleanliness and discipline among the soldiers (52). As information and goods "moved back and forth between Washington, the military outpost, and the most distant households of the United States," women became the voices of cleanliness in the interest of their families (53). Helen Campbell wrote in 1897 in *Household Economics: A Course of Lectures in the School of Economics of the University of Wisconsin*: "to keep the world clean—this is the one great task for women" (59).

In these accounts white, middle-class women not only were assigned a major role as the guardians of domestic health, but also, as I have argued in this book, themselves became associated with the unclean. "Sanitary products" or "sanitary napkins" can still be found at the rear of pharmacy shops next to incontinence aids, their brand names attesting to their unspoken, hidden presence: Whisper, Invisible, Slims, and Ultrathins. The naming of these products as "sanitary" pays homage to the connection between the germ theory of disease and the resultant sanitary crusade against dangerous enemies within. A tampon product called Meds marketed by Modess in 1946 asserted that the tampons were "made of 'surgical cotton' and 'hygienically sealed in individual containers'" (Houppert 1999, 15–16). All manner of sprays, powders, wipes, and deodorants can also be purchased "to give extra reassurance, especially during warm weather and menstruation." The advertising states that these "intimate feminine hygiene" products contain antibacterial agents designed to "absorb moisture and neutralize odors . . . to keep [women] feeling clean, fresh, dry and confident." There is no equivalent marketing directed toward men's bodies, their products being sold under the generic banner of "toiletries."

Domestic Hygiene

It is women who are positioned as battling against invisible germs and diseases in the home. This was made clear to me when, after the birth of my daughter, I received a free gift bag from a leading Australian shopping chain. Included in the bag were a number of free samples, the majority of which were cleaning agents: a spray can of air freshener to "eliminate nasty toilet odors" and two separate antibacterial cleaners for the kitchen and the bathroom. Now that I was a mother, the accompanying brochure instructed me, "proper cleaning is an important part of maintaining a healthy home for your family." By using the antibacterial cleaners, it was my role to prevent cross-contamination between the bathroom and kitchen. As Cowan notes: "Cleaning the bathroom sink [is] not just cleaning, but an exercise for the maternal instincts, protecting the family from disease" (1976, 151).[13]

The positioning of women in the home as agents of health and hygiene was epitomized among the participants by Grace, whose house had been described by the community nurse as "immaculate" and "neat as a pin." In the home that she shared with her husband and teenage son, Grace showed me the rows of tins and neatly labeled jars in her pantry cupboards, and endless handwritten notes about planned recipes. The one bookcase in the kitchen/dining area was filled with cookbooks, some that she had used when training as a cordon bleu chef in England. With her orange-colored hands (from eating too many carrots, she said), Grace showed me her treasured cookbooks, including one handed down through the generations from her grandmother to her own mother and then to her.[14] A weighty, dark red, leather-bound, 2,500-page volume titled *Mrs Beeton's Book of Household Management*, this was a "guide to cookery in all branches" and included seventy-four chapters pertaining to tasks associated with "womenly duties," such as "mistress and servant, hostess and guest, home doctor, sick nursing, and the nursery." (Grace had the 1907 edition; the book was originally published in 1861.)[15] Its final pages included a detailed section on hygiene and contagious diseases, drawing heavily on the miasmatic theory of disease and germ theory. Ways of countering sickness included "sufficient supply of pure air," "pure water" (rainwater in particular), "frequent washing and clean utensils" (Beeton 1907, 1823–1903). *Mrs Beeton's Book of Household Management* was far more than a cookbook; it was an instructional manual for women.[16]

Even though Grace found the instructions antiquated and we laughed at their fussiness, she practiced many of the enduring rules of hygiene and order in her own home. Surfaces in her kitchen were kept hygienically clean. She washed her hands after touching uncooked meats, after reading the newspaper, and after a shopping trip. When her anorexia was at its worst, she would take weeks to plan meals for her family, taking notes from each cookbook as to what to prepare. Her attention to the details of household management so preoccupied her every thought that she would sometimes take cookbooks to bed at night to read.

Many other participants displayed and spoke about their meticulous attendance to household cleanliness—the arbitrary rules of household maintenance. In fridges I saw cans of diet drink perfectly lined up with their labels facing front; clothes hung in order on the line—a row of socks, a row of pants, a row of stockings, each row hung with color-matching pegs. Towels and underpants were repeatedly soaked in the antibacterial washing detergent Nappy San to remove and kill germs. Bathrooms were spotless, and kitchens belied their functions, as there were rarely dishes on the sink and no visible signs of food or cutlery/crockery. Bettina laughed about the times that she used to wash the laundry sink, taps, washing machine, clothes pegs, and clothesline, all before actually doing the washing. Then she'd have to wash her hands "in case of germs." My initial reaction to her house (in which she had lived alone for four years) in my field notes captured the sense of order and cleanliness:

> She offered me a seat and said: "Would you like to see my house and then we'll have a coffee" . . . as she wanted to show me her house before "it got mucked up." She told me how she had spent a good few hours tidying in anticipation of my arrival—washing floors and putting things in their place. There was hardly any indication that this unit was lived in (in the sense of any evidence of everyday household mess or

> activities)—very few personal mementos of Bettina (except the glass cabinet of dolls and the toy baby bassinette wrapped in plastic)—no toiletries in the bathroom, no papers lying about, no books, no photographs, no pictures on any of the walls, nothing on any of the dressing tables—only two lonely pairs of her shoes next to her queen size bed. She later "confessed" that she slept in the single bed in the spare room as her mother had suggested it would mean less sheets to wash. The flat was quite clinical in some ways because it was so ordered, neat, and "clean."

Some participants were reticent about inviting me to their homes, and this reticence was often related to their homes being unclean (or the presence of family members). Rita and I usually met in a public park, but as the weather began to chill with the onset of winter, she invited me to the unit that she shared with Daisy, her dog. As I swung my car into her driveway I saw the curtain of the front window pull back, and she was out the front door and ready to go before I could step out of the car. She asked if we could go to a coffee shop at a nearby shopping center, as her house, she said, was "wallowing in [her] own filth."

The first time Natalia invited me to her home, she explained how she had been cleaning for most of the previous night, laughing that it was a good excuse not to have to sleep, as sleeping slowed "the body's metabolism down and burnt less calories." Every time I visited she would allow me to view a different part of her home. On this occasion she showed me the kitchen, inside her fridge and cupboards, and her garden. As I entered the front door I noticed the Japanese slippers inside the entrance and asked if she would like me to take my shoes off (she would). She took me through to the brightly lit, open plan kitchen. On the opposite wall over the kitchen bench was a glass cabinet that displayed a number of miniature Japanese scenes; a tea ceremony, musical instruments, miniature people made out of paper, miniature figures of animals representing the years, and a small book to explain it all. We marveled at the meticulous attention to detail in each case. All surfaces were completely bare—there were no dishes on the sink, or any visible signs of food or cans or anything to do with cooking. She fetched a flashlight and shone it into the huge back yard. Down the central path was a line of pots, mainly miniature roses which she had pruned that day. Under the veranda were pots of camellias, to the left was the Japanese section (sacred bamboo and succulents), against the fence were more pots, and there was also a line around the bottom of the caravan and the large tin shed (poor man's orchids). All the plants were in pots and grouped according to species. Back in the kitchen Natalia asked if I would like to look in the cupboards, and she opened the one nearest the outer door. It was neatly stacked with food items, arranged from tallest at the back to smallest at the front, and again grouped and categorized into similar food items.

This overwhelming desire for cleanliness and order was central to the symbolic rituals of purification described earlier in the chapter. By maintaining an ordered environment, participants themselves felt cleaner, as Tamara suggested: "It's just wanting everything to be clean and perfect and new almost—how I want myself to be." As already mentioned, her bodily washing was a way of alleviating the guilt, shame, and disgust she felt with her own body after being raped. Tamara and many other others used hygienic practices to disconnect themselves from things they found disgusting and out of place: foods, bodily processes, memories, experiences, and emotions.

(A)voiding Emotions

While the discovery of microbes appealed to reason and was based upon scientifically proven facts about disease and bacteria, an emotional imperative was also central to the efficacy of hygiene. This imperative relied on arousing feelings of anxiety, guilt, fear, and shame about dirt. Attempts to transform cleanliness into a moral issue were presented in advertisements, school curricula, and household economy texts, where "disorder and lack of cleanliness [were said to] cause a sort of suffering in the mistress of the house" (Forty 1986, 169).[17] The design of household items (such as white baths and refrigerators) in the 1920s began to embody these virtues, "warning of the consequences of neglecting health and cleanliness which ranged from emotional rejection by loved ones to social ostracism, illness, death and national downfall" (170). Removing dirt went hand in hand with erasing these associated emotions, for if dirt was removed and objects put in place and ordered, then fear and guilt concerning disease and domestic duties was alleviated. It was precisely these emotions of anxiety, guilt, fear, and shame that circulated in participants' narratives and everyday lives.

These emotive aspects of hygiene continue to play an integral part in its logic, and we all often use dirt or cleanliness metaphors when speaking of emotion. Talking about intimate details was often characterized by participants as "airing dirty laundry," "coming clean," "like having a big vomit" or a purging.[18] Estelle described the therapeutic device of talking with psychiatrists as "spilling her guts"; it was a method of "getting it out, of coming clean."[19] Talking as purging is also a common practice in Christian religions (and on popular television chat shows), where the confession is designed to absolve one's sins.

Speaking, however, was not always an available route for coming clean. In the introduction to this book I describe some participants' inability to speak about certain issues, an inability compounded by their social withdrawal.

For those like Tanya, anorexia took away "all forms of emotional expression," including singing, listening to music, and writing poetry. She describes herself as being "really withdrawn from everyone and I didn't see any of my friends, and while I'd be home with my family a lot I wouldn't talk with them or interact with them in any way." "Anorexia," she explained, "stops you from being able to connect." It also made her feel empty and pure. "I always had the numb feeling inside," she said. "I never allowed myself to feel anything and if anything went wrong in my life that might possibly upset me, I just pushed it away and convinced myself that I was really strong and could just deal with these things."

"Why would you want to push away emotions?" I asked. "What is it about emotions that makes you want to do that?"

"I guess just not wanting to feel. Nobody wants to feel pain. I think it's trying to avoid getting hurt."[20]

Fluids That Carry Emotions

Participants who could not avoid painful emotions or feelings of disgust and dirt described other avenues of (a)voiding. The ways in which people with anorexia metaphorically spilled their guts—absolved disgust and shame—was literally by spilling their guts, by vomiting. Emotions were also purged by taking laxatives to induce diarrhea, excessively exercising to sweat, taking diuretics to rapidly increase urine output, spitting food out, washing bodies, and bloodletting. It was by way of fluids that emotions were released from their bodies, as Estelle explained: "I didn't really care about having diarrhea because I felt better afterwards. . . . I used to think—it's really stupid, but it's a metaphor—and I used to think it got rid of all the shit inside me. I felt like a bad person so I felt better. It was a way of flushing out the bad things.

"What were the bad things you were flushing out?" I asked Estelle.

"I thought I was really greedy and selfish and bad," she said. I was sometimes punishing myself—like if I ate something bad I would take more laxatives than I usually did to make myself feel better."

"And when you say 'better,' " I clarified, "cleaner, not so dirty."

It is useful to clarify the way in which I use the term "emotion" in my discussion, for anthropological studies of this topic differ in their orientation. In his comprehensive review of theorizing emotion in anthropology, Leavitt (1996) highlights the disembodied characterizations that some authors suggest. Lutz and White, for example, argue that emotion is not an "internal state" (1986, 408); Lynch writes that "emotions are not passions" (1990, 10); and others, such as Solomon, suggest that "an emotion is not a feeling (or a set of feelings), but an interpretation" (1984, 248). Lutz and Abu-Lughod in their edited *Language and the Politics of Emotion* consider emotion a discourse rather than a felt experience. They argue that "rather than seeing them [emotions] as expressive vehicles, we must understand emotional discourses as pragmatic acts and communicative performances" (11).

Two incisive critiques argue against a discursive approach to emotion. While acknowledging the attempt to break through "the prison house of language" created by structuralism and certain strands of semiotics, Desjarlais criticizes the approach for discussing "everything save what poetic discourses themselves seem to speak about: most commonly, profound experiences of grief, sadness and pain; . . . any reference to emotion implies, by definition, something 'felt'" (1992, 100–101). Leavitt similarly attacks Lutz and Abu-Lughod 1990 for their language of construction, arguing that terms such as "language," "speech," and "discourse" negate the "bodily, expressive, or personal" forms of emotion (1996, 523). Both Leavitt and Desjarlais point to the interwoven relationship of language and bodily experience. Meaning and practice, Desjarlais states, should be studied "in tandem, mapping the nature of meaning in practice and the social practice of meaning" (1992, 101).

In agreeing with these critiques, my understanding of emotion involves both meaning and feeling, for as Leavitt suggests, emotion words are precisely the ones we use when we do not want to be forced into a choice of either/or categories (1996, 523). In an analytical sense then, emotions are fluid, for they cross conceptual boundaries; they connect meaning and feeling and dualist constructions of mind and body. They are also fluid in terms of embodiment, because they similarly transgress bodily boundaries by the very nature of their flow. In light of my discussion of purging, I extend Desjarlais's and Leavitt's arguments to suggest that bodily fluids carry emotions, and in this fieldwork, specifically emotions of disgust, guilt, and shame.

The positioning of emotion within an experiential rather than a discursive approach has parallels with the overarching themes of this book. Take a moment to consider the example of Estelle just related. If one were to apply a discursive approach to her purging practices, then ideas of containment and individualism—the discursive constructions of the self—would be the focus. This is precisely the interpretation that Malson takes in her discussion of purging (despite her poststructuralist claims): "Within the framework of a discourse of individualism identity is produced as something internal, and 'purging' obliterates this internality, producing an emptied, voided self; a subjectivity that resonates with those constructions of the self as an identity-less, empty shell" (1998, 168).

By focusing not on categories of self or individualism but on the actual fluids that move between them, fluids are shown not to be simply a means to an end but to play a central role in purging practices. Purging fluids is what transformed experience for participants, for the bodily fluids of vomit, diarrhea, sweat, urine, spit, and blood (including menstrual blood) carry disgust away from the body. Fluids are pivotal because of their ability to transform relationships, to carry and move emotion.

The connection between fluids and emotion is not surprising. The etymology of "emotion" points to the centrality of movement and motion in its meaning: "agitation, tumult," "move the feelings of," "after *mouvoir*, motion," "causing movement" (Onions 1966, 310; see also Epstein 1993, 100). The central role of emotion in human agency, as Telfer notes, is its intimate connection to movement (1998, 271). Kapferer takes a similar view: "Emotions are forms of the expression of the fluid motion . . . of human beings in the world" (1997, 223). Emotions are a fundamental part of relatedness, for people can be moved by emotions and can use them to form connections and disconnections.

Participants often used metaphors involving fluids to emphasize the emotional qualities of their experiences; they described "bursting into tears," "spilling their guts," things that "made them sick" (metaphorically), and "pouring their hearts out." More generally, bodily fluids that carry emotions included tears (of happiness and sadness), fluids associated with waste that carry disgust and dirt (as described earlier), and those that, when out of place, carry danger (blood). Yet, people with anorexia also described expelling these fluids as a cleansing of emotion, as we have seen. Purging did not leave them without an identity or as empty shells as Malson suggests; instead, it cleansed and transformed their embodied states.

Out, Damned Spot! Spilling Blood and Guilt

The most dramatic method of purging emotion was the cutting of skin to let blood. Sonya, who had left anorexia, told me: "There's a lot who do it, and a lot won't tell you. They'll cut on the soles of their feet and they won't tell anybody. But they will tell another anorexic who does the same thing." These practices are known to psychiatrists as self-mutilation or self-injury, distinct from but not dissimilar to bloodletting (see Favazza 1996). Although the techniques of opening the skin are different, both place importance on the symbolism of blood and the emotional release that accompanies its loss.

The practice of bloodletting is a rare phenomenon among those diagnosed with eating disorders. One psychiatrist noted that in his clinical work with eating-disordered patients over the past fifteen years, he had "seen it only once, in a nurse with chronic anorexia nervosa" (Vandereycken 1993, 851). Bloodletting refers to "venipuncture or insertion of intravenous cannulae," that is, small tubes, to let blood from the body (Parkin and Eagles 1993, 246). In reported cases it is often those who have access to medical supplies and proficiency in venipuncture, such as medical students, nurses, and doctors, who practice bloodletting. One medical student with bulimia nervosa regularly let her blood because "it afforded her a 'release' from feelings of anger and tension. As she lost blood she felt 'distanced, euphoric and satisfied.' She equated it with the feeling she derived from vomiting after a binge, but felt much less guilty about bloodletting" (247). Another clinician similarly describes bloodletting as a purging behavior, a "stress-reducing behavior" (Cosman 1986, 1188).

Although no participants bloodlet by venipuncture, I was aware that four released blood by cutting their skin with glass, scissors, knives, and razor blades. In the park one day, Rita, who always wore long skirts and long-sleeved shirts, showed me scars from Stanley knife cuts: "I've done my arms and both thighs. It sounds revolting, but I actually like to see the slash. . . . I like to see the blood coming out, I like to see it pouring out." Sitting on her living room couch with towels under her arms, she would make deep cuts in her legs and left arm to get "rid of something that is putrid, the ugliness and badness in me. "To me it's like an elimination, like a purging, getting rid of something really bad. It's like polluted—it's bad blood, as I call it. I want it all to ooze out of me and be gone. It's satisfying at the time, but the next day of course you feel like a total prat and an idiot and then you take weeks to bloody heal up again, but at the time of doing it there's some sort of release, some sort of purging thing going on there . . . get out of me. It's like vomiting blood except you do it through your cuts."

Amanda also wanted to remove the "badness in her body," "to do something bad with [her] bad self."[21] "I don't know why I do it, except for some reason it helps. I don't know if these are my words or someone else's words, but it is a bit of a release—it relieves me in some ways."

"What are you getting rid of?" I asked. I noticed that she was clenching her fists.

"I guess it's kind of anger at myself or hatred at myself and at the world and at my lot in the world," Amanda said, "and this happens when I'm really depressed so it's not like how I am now, it's a lot different. It's that really wound-up feeling you get in your chest. . . . The blood is like you can see it coming—you can see the anger coming out."

It could be argued that the metaphors used to describe this release of anger simply draw upon dichotomous constructions of the self and body. Desjarlais, in reflecting on the display of emotions among the Yolma, states that "the idea that unvented anger builds up and then needs to be 'let out' to avoid an explosion stems from the mechanistic 'hydraulic' theory of emotional expression common to several Western and non-Western philosophies of the self" (1992, 116). In positioning bodily fluids as carriers of emotion, this analysis moves away from a focus on structures and explores the ways in which meanings move between categories, as I have noted. It is literally the movement of fluids that was transformational.

For Sonya, it was the movement of blood out of her body and the smearing or painting of the fluid onto surfaces (including her face) that was transformative. As a visual artist, she sometimes used her own blood as a medium to create pictorial narratives of her disgust and distress. In her white-tiled bathroom she would cut her forearms, upper chest, and calves to "stop [herself] feeling like a pressure cooker," to release the guilt and anger. The cutting itself was not painful: "You dissociate from your body, you can't feel your body, it feels numb, and you cut and it feels like cutting through butter. It is purging. All that guilt and all that anger is just trickling out. You have to see it, and I think part of it is like in our culture what blood represents too—you know it's the lifeblood, it's red, it represents violence. It's just like you see it coming out and it's all that anger pouring out and that's why you don't want to clean it up. And then later I did—" she laughed weakly, "this is kinda funny—I did paintings with the blood, yeah."

"What sort of paintings?" I asked.

"Paintings. I'd take the blood and paint with it—either with my fingers or with the patio brush."

"And what would you be painting?"

"Oh, some abstract and some figures and some are things out of my psyche," Sonya said. "I'll show you them." She went on to describe the feeling that motivated these paintings. "At the time that I did the painting in blood, I really believed that I was responsible for all the abuse. I felt at the time that it was the female flesh on my body that attracted the men to me for sex at age eleven. No matter how much I starved myself or cut at myself to punish the flesh and let out the blood, it was never enough. I would not have been satisfied until all that was left was bone. Bone is strong and carries no female flesh or semblance of femininity. No male would ever want me. But like Lady MacBeth, no matter how much she washed and scrubbed, it [the guilt and disgust] never went away." One of the paintings Sonya painted with her blood in fact depicted Lady MacBeth washing the guilt away.

Hovering at the Borders

Purification, as Sonya suggests, was not a straightforward process. These practices were only momentarily effective, for the impure, as Kristeva argues, can never be completely removed: "getting rid of [the abject] is out of the question; . . . one does not get rid of the impure" (1982, 28). The closeness of disgust to the body, the sense that it never goes away, was a common experience. Purging practices were shrouded in secrecy, characterized as "a terrible dirty secret" and "the most disgusting habit" of those of which participants were ashamed.[22]

I asked Linda, "Do you remember how you felt when you were vomiting, when you were purging yourself?" She became distressed as she described her experience: "Glad, very glad, but it was hell, it was really, really—it was just hell." She began to cry and I asked if we should stop. "No," she said, "it's okay, it's just that it disgusts me, it completely disgusts me but I had to get the food out of me." Disgust and shame, as Probyn suggests, are coiled together in the body; they are powerful affects that need to be "reintegrated into thinking about corporeal politics" (2000, 125). Participants not only talked of how shameful purging was to them, but also described the shame of being caught. Daily purging in shared houses meant that they had to have excuses at the ready or feign innocence. The most common tactics of concealment were pleading regular bouts of "gastro" (gastroenteritis) or acting surprised when the plumbing blocked again. Like the tactics of *la perruque* in the outwitting of staff and family, hiding and lying about purging was a common practice. Even those who lived alone would take precautions against unwanted intruders. Lara, who lived alone in a small council flat, described the tension associated with her purging: "I even get paranoid that someone's going to telephone while I'm doing it and know what I'm doing. I used to leave the phone off the hook so nobody would phone and disrupt me."

"What would happen if someone did walk in or interrupt you?" I asked.

"Nobody knows except for [one close friend] really that I still do it," Lara said. "I also dread the doorbell going, but I'll just pretend I'm out. The phone rang once and I actually answered it and it was my friend and I said, 'I'm in a meeting, I'll phone you back in an hour!'" She laughed. "I thought, I cannot be interrupted, I have to get rid of this food."

The alternative framework for exploring the connections between the individual pathologies of anorexia and obsessive-compulsive disorders presented here rejects understanding the range of behaviors as symptomatic of a comorbid disorder, as another layering of illness, and demonstrates instead the logic of practice in which participants felt compelled to cleanse themselves. The experiences of abjection of food, bodies, and experiences described in the last three chapters suggest that many of the purging practices associated with anorexia are concerned with the casting out of that which is disgusting. These practices include not only the more common eliminations of purging and laxative use, but also washing, scrubbing, and sanitizing particular parts of bodies and environments.

An overwhelming desire for cleanliness and order were central to the symbolic rituals of purification described earlier in the chapter. Heretofore, purity has been linked with analyses of anorexia only through religious discourses of asceticism. Garrett (1992, 1998), for example, in her Durkheimian studies, suggests that "anorexia can be interpreted as a purity ritual [in which] anthropological theories of asceticism, ritual and religion offer a way of conceptualizing anorexia and recovery as linked stages in a profoundly social transformation of the individual self" (1998, 58). Purity, as this ethnography has demonstrated, is not solely located in these domains but intersects with a number of other fields: medicine, nutrition, sexuality, and ideas of the clean, proper, and virtuous body. Hygiene is a central field through which all these logics of practices resonate.

Everyday practices of hygiene enabled the women in this research to disconnect themselves from that which they found disgusting and out of place: certain foods, bodily processes, relationships, memories, experiences, and emotions. Hygienic practices transformed relations of disgust into states of asexuality, asceticism, and asepsis. These were not simply "profound transformations of the individual self," but more importantly, profound transformations of social relations.

8

Reimagining Anorexia

The aim of this book has been to provide a new approach to the phenomenon of anorexia. In my discussion of anorexia there is one player that I have consciously relegated to the background: the media. As I argued in the introduction, I did not wish to reproduce the discursive explanation of anorexia as a "reading disorder" and tried to steer away from media representations of anorexia. I anticipated that in focusing on participants' everyday worlds, my fieldwork would be led away from the disembodied textual analyses that have already been extensively explored in the eating disorder literature. As my fieldwork progressed, however, I came to realize that to disengage from the power of these representations would be a grave methodological error.

This realization was unavoidable when, toward the end of my research for the book, parts of it were broadcast and printed in the national and international media. It is these very particular representations of anorexia, and their relationship to psychiatry and anthropology, that I address here. In examining the underpinning framings of these characterizations, the major analytical strands of this book come together. Ironically, my conclusions are situated in that which I initially tried to ignore—the intertwined relationship of ethnography and the media.

Turning Up the White Noise

The relationship between the media and ethnographic enquiry is problematized by Ortner, who broadens the term "media" to "public culture" in order to generate a more inclusive approach to representational systems. Public culture, she argues, includes "all the bodies of images, claims, and representations created to speak to and about the actual people who live in the US: all of the products of art and entertainment (film, television, books, etc.), as well as all of the texts of information and analysis (all forms of journalism and academic production)" (1999, 55). It is through these pervasive and taken-for-granted representations that "lifestyles, habits, tastes and attitudes are everywhere, and inescapably before us. . . . Who [then] can presume to step 'outside' of it? Its ideas and assumptions are everywhere, and not least in our own minds" (Ehrenreich 1990, cited in ibid.). The same can be claimed about knowledges and representations of anorexia.

Examples of this inescapable relationship were the anonymous flyers that appeared during my fieldwork with increasing regularity: "Lose weight fast"; "Lose 15 kilograms in 3 weeks"; "Lose weight now, ask me how."[1] At first these advertisements annoyed me and I tried to ignore them; they smacked of the insidious commercialism that flourishes around the weight-loss industry and get-rich-quick schemes. But I couldn't ignore this pervasive "white noise" of fieldwork (see also Marcus 1998, 96). Their appearances became more intrusive and significant. Returning to my car following a hospital visit, I found a flyer stuck to the windscreen. When I was unchaining my bike late one night from a lamppost outside a community support service for people with eating disorders, I looked up and there, glued to the pole, was a flyer. After poring over the minute details of food-packaging labels in a supermarket, a participant and I returned to the car to find a weight-loss advertisement flapping under the windscreen wiper.

The flyers acted as a forcible reminder of the connections between the fields in which participants and I moved, between institutions, community organizations, public spaces, and people's homes. Media representations were ubiquitous in each. While waiting in hospital corridors and waiting rooms, I picked up women's magazines and read stories about movie stars' weight losses/successes, and sometimes stories of someone's "battle with an eating disorder." At Lane Cove a young woman recovering from anorexia leapt across the cushions of the lounge to turn off the television advertisement for a multinational weight-loss consortium. Amanda would while away hours on the bed program by cutting out stories about weight loss (and recipes) in magazines to add to her already voluminous collection at home. The plethora of such media provided community groups with so much ammunition against stereotypes of women and anorexia that one community organization filled a bulletin board at its main office entrance with an ever-changing array of offending clippings.[2]

These were the fields in which people traveled, part of their everyday worlds and experiences. To ignore the interconnections between experiences and objects, between people and places, would be to explore only part of their worlds. My field sites, like the everyday worlds of participants, were not pristine, bounded, or contained. People moved back and forth between a number of fields, each field enmeshed in and generating its own representations, knowledges, and powers. And in these fields, people were always "caught in fragments of representational systems" (Chakrabarty 1994, 100).

Chakrabarty's statement was brought home to me during the writing-up phase of this book when a journalist from my home university's paper requested an interview (and photograph) about my research. Intense media interest followed publication of this story. I was inundated with phone calls from national and international radio and television presenters and print media journalists (including magazine editors and newspaper journalists). Many of those involved in the visual media requested interviews with women from this project, and when I pressed them, it was clear that they wanted images of emaciated bodies to fuel their stories. Even though I denied these requests, one television interview drew images from its archives and displayed semi-naked pictures of starved young women as the backdrop to my research. It was thus not only the participants who were caught in representational systems, but also my own ethnographic research.

Primitivizing Anorexia

A media story that illustrates the relationship between this ethnography and public culture covered two pages in a major Australian newspaper. Headlined "Tribal Starvation" and "The Secret Suffering," the story outlined how "new research has discovered a surprising subculture among people with eating disorders," claiming that "within the inner sanctum of eating disorders lies a maze of cults" and announcing that "you are either part of the strange starvation tribe—or you are not" (*The Age*, June 22, 2001). Two black-and-white images were used in conjunction with the story. The first was of two shadowy figures facing forward (one clearly a woman, from her mode of dress); both were faceless and had willowy bodies. The other image was of a young woman standing in front of a mirror, her frowning face reflecting her dissatisfaction with her distorted image. The mirror was similar to those found in a sideshow at any carnival or traveling show (indeed there is a warped image of a Ferris wheel in the mirror). This oft repeated idea of distorted body image clearly points to the ways in which this women's experience of her own body is at odds with how other people view her. Her perceptions (in this case her gaze) are deemed distorted and irrational.

What the text and images of this story play with are key concepts of primitivism: representations of difference, distance, and otherness. Primitivism, as writers like Torgovnick (1990), Clifford (1990), and Lucas and Barrett (1995) suggest, is "a body of ideas, images and vocabularies about cultural others" that has been used to construct and imagine otherness and identity throughout a variety of fields (Lucas and Barrett 1995, 289). Lucas and Barrett demonstrate how psychiatry is implicated in this particular configuration of knowledge. They examine three principal (but by no means definitive) subject areas of cross-cultural psychiatry—*amok*, the therapeutic potential of traditional society, and the shaman—arguing that "psychiatric primitivism" has been invoked as an explanatory framework in each. In accounts of *amok*, for example, it is claimed that "people in less developed societies exhibit a "passivity of mind and an unpreparedness for sudden decision and action, reducing them to 'primitive' defense reactions such as fright" (Kiev 1972, 73, cited in ibid., 299). Similarly, shamans have been represented by two opposing types of psychiatric primitivism, through both barbaric images of madness (as a malevolent trickster and fraud) and Arcadian images of healing (a visionary or seer). In all these schemas, images of society, person, and mental illness converge, so that each comes to signify the other. These "clichéd categories of primitivism" underpin cross-cultural psychiatry's understanding of mental illness (313).

Primitivism is not confined to representations of the Other, for it is also fundamentally concerned with the ways in which the self is imagined. It is, as Lucas and Barrett argue, "an essentially reflexive tool by which the West comes to understand itself. In the process it constructs the Other as an exotic from a distant land, or as a threatening presence concealed within the Western self" (ibid.). These types of constructions, as Clifford suggests, are "a way of coming to know and contain that which is forbidden, marked off and tabooed in our own society, in this case 'madness'" (1990, 142). In terms of psychiatry, primitivism is thus "one of the principal means of understanding mental illness in Western psychiatry" (Lucas and Barrett 1995, 314).

It was the barbaric form of primitivism that the print media continually drew upon in its characterizations of my research. This is not to suggest that the journalists concerned were familiar with the history or epistemologies of psychiatry. Rather it points to the wider circulation of primitivist ideas within what Ortner has defined as "public culture." Moreover, I suggest that it was the particular configuration of my research—of anthropology, psychiatry, and anorexia—that proved irresistible to such primitivist characterizations. The images and words used to describe my research are synonymous with barbaric primitivism. Compare barbaric primitivism's "stranger from an exotic land," part of an "inchoate tribe," and "bound by superstition and irrationality" (Lucas and Barrett 1995, 290, 296) with the media's treatment of anorexia: "tribal," "maze of cults," "strange," "subculture" (*The Age*, June 22, 2001); "mysterious starving condition" (*The Advertiser*, June 5, 2001); "dangerous" (*Daily Telegraph*, June 5, 2001); and "cult-like" (*Canberra Times*, June 5, 2001). Primitivism was the story's hook to engage the reader, an invitation to be fascinated and horrified by "tribal starvation." The message was that people (and predominantly women) with anorexia may be familiar to us, but they are most remarkably not like us by their strange desire to waste away.

Despite the reflexive turn within anthropology (and social sciences and humanities more generally), the relevance of these debates has not entered public culture with the same fervor. In the public domain anthropology remains trapped within a primitivist understanding, as a discipline that continues to represent the Other. Psychiatry, similarly, is characterized in public culture as a marginal stream of medicine that deals with the other of madness. The media representations of my work engaged with the simple dichotomies that primitivism provides, unable (or unwilling) to engage with the complexities, subtleties, and ambiguities that anorexia might present.

The Othering of Abjection

It could be argued that there are parallels between primitivism and abjection, that the language of Kristeva's abject is synonymous with the language of primitivism. Both, for example, are concerned with difference and desire, self and other, familiarity and strangeness, horror and fascination. These are the precise tropes from which I distanced myself in the introduction to this book, where I criticized simplistic reductions of anorexia to carnivalesque image of thinness, horror, fascination, and death. Certainly, as Lechte suggests, there is an "emotionally charged fascination with abjection. Horror and fascination are intertwined" (1990, 167). There is a danger that abjection could be taken as simply another way of representing people with anorexia as primitive other.

While this ethnography is as much a representation of anorexia as the media story presented earlier, its modes of representation are entirely different. It is important to reemphasise these differences, for they underpin the central arguments of this book and highlight the significant contribution of ethnography to this domain of research.

Although primitivism and abjection use a similar wording of difference and otherness, their usage is framed by different epistemologies that result in completely different meanings. My strategy was not to erase problematic terms such as "self" or "other," but to rethink their relationship ethnographically, as I suggested in chapter 4. I have done this by approaching these terms through a concept of relatedness, by examining the ways in which "selves become [and unbecome] . . . within a matrix of relations with others" (Ingold 1991, 367). This matrix is, in Bourdieu's sense, a field of social relationships in which relations unfold and enfold in the processes of social life (ibid.). People with anorexia often experienced these processes as abject, for they conflated and transgressed representational categories that constructed their social worlds.

The constructions that frame primitivism rely on static dualisms that fix the separate categories of self and other into an either/or schema. This fixing serves to create autonomous categories that stand in hierarchical opposition to one another. Civilized, for example, is conceptualized as present and near, whereas primitive is located in historical time and in faraway places. As Fabian (1983) has shown, a certain politics of time and space is evoked in primitivist constructions to distance others, despite their contemporary presence.

While Kristeva's concept of abjection uses the language of self and other, it is not dualistic, for it is concerned with the movement within and in between these categories. In extending abjection into an ethnographic domain, this book has highlighted the relational aspects of anorexia (with oneself, with others, and with objects). Chapters 4 through 7 described the relationships that people with anorexia had with each other, family members, and friends, with different types of foods, with their bodies, and with spaces. What was striking about these relationships was that they were experienced as abject: as simultaneously threatening, desired and disgusting. That which is abject is not trapped in dualisms or reduced to oppositions. On the contrary, what is abject is in between, ambiguous, and composite. Abjection is thus contrary to dualist concepts because it undermines and threatens that which is separate. As such, abjection is fundamentally concerned with the complexities and contradictions of relatedness.

The dualist categories of self and other pay homage to the notion of an autonomous and unchanging subject or self. As an ongoing process, Kristeva's understanding of self-identification involves a new model of otherness within the subject. Recall the descriptions of my own experiences of alterity through pregnancy (chapter 3). Pregnancy problematizes the concept of the autonomous self, for "the maternal body is the very embodiment of alterity-within. It cannot be neatly divided into subject and object" (Oliver 1993, 4). While a discussion (and critique) of Kristeva's problematic account of "becoming mother" is outside the purviews of this book, my own experience of pregnancy in the field highlighted the very notions of self-identity and difference that abjection holds in tension.

Participants experienced this "alterity-within" through the personification of anorexia. This ethnography has described how they entered into and developed intimate relationships with anorexia; it became a friend, an angel, or the devil in disguise. Anorexia had the attributes of an abusive lover. It was, as Elise said, "very seductive; it draws you in, it's like a safe relationship. . . . It's like an abusive relationship, but it's very difficult to get out of and you can go back so many times." These constant struggles of separation and seduction are, Kristeva argues, integral to the process of self-identification, of acknowledging and confronting the other within the self. This confrontation is the substance of abjection, the experience of a "violent, clumsy breaking away, with the constant risk of falling back under the sway of a power as securing as it stifling" (Kristeva 1982, 13).

The relationships that participants had were never static but, like any social relationships, were constantly shifting and transforming. As Estelle's account of her "recovery phase" highlighted, relationships in treatment settings were complex sites of negotiation, not only with other inpatients but also with staff members (see chapter 4). These were places where her identity was performed, constructed, and deconstructed in multiple ways. Although Estelle was legitimated as a patient through the diagnosis of anorexia, there was an entirely different level of legitimation being played out among other inpatients. To the ward staff, Estelle had anorexia, but to other inpatients with anorexia she was outside anorexia because of her desire to overcome it. Estelle found this multiple identification problematic, in that she was caught between the authoring of competing forces. In short, the narratives described in this book reconceptualize the discursive production of self and other as relational rather than oppositional.

The final difference between abjection and primitivism relates to differing experiences of self and other within fields. As I have argued, primitivism works on the premise of a clear-cut relationship between self and other, of the distant gaze upon the object of display. What is objectified evokes the spectacle of primitivism, be it Kafka's hunger artist behind the bars of the performing cage, static displays behind glass in museums or art galleries, or photographs of other locations and peoples. The distance reinforces the conceptual relationship between self and other. Unlike the gaze, abjection is located in visceral and sensual bodies. It may be evoked through the gaze, but it is fundamentally experienced through the perceptual modalities that evoke emotive responses: taste, touch, and smell. It is not disembodied, objectified, and distant, but felt and close. Experiences of anorexia are thus not concerned simply with body image—with how one looks—but also with experiences that one feels.

In focusing on the embodiment of anorexia, this ethnography has not represented participants as objects for others to gaze upon, but has positioned their experiences as central. These experiences were grounded in relatedness. In their everyday lives, participants maneuvered in and out, between and within a set of indeterminate relations. Jackson argues that the experience of constant maneuvering between self and other (rather than the terms themselves) is "indicative of the way human experience vacillates between a sense of ourselves as subjects and as objects; in effect, making us feel sometimes that we are world makers, sometimes that we are merely made by the world" (1996, 21). Experiences of anorexia are clearly not one thing or another, but oscillate between categories.

The emphasis on relatedness and abjection throughout this ethnography has taken the arguments on a very different course from that of a discursive reading of anorexia. Discursive representations such as primitivism bear no relationship to people's experiences of anorexia. Participants were not part of a strange starvation tribe, "exotic being[s], unpredictable and governed by instincts and emotions" (Lucas and Barrett 1995, 289). On the contrary, I have argued that experiences of anorexia draw directly from people's habitus, from their everyday relationships with people, places, food, bodies, sexuality, and gender relations. For a variety of reasons, participants began to experience these aspects of their lives as dirty and disgusting. They turned to the cultural frameworks of purity and hygiene to cleanse themselves and their environments. Hygienic practices ensured that purity could be attained in all its ideological and functional facets. Bodies could become clean through practices of purging, washing, and eating only clean foods, disengaging from the messiness of sexuality and sexual relationships, and sanitizing and ordering environments.

This process, however, did not completely remove dirt and disgust, for purging was only a temporary alleviation of disgust. What was cast out could never be completely removed but, as Kristeva suggests, hovered close to the body. Experiences of anorexia are replete with ambiguity and misrecognition, as in Hornbacher's succinct description:

> It is, at the most basic level, a bundle of deadly contradictions: a desire for power that strips you of all power. A gesture of strength that divests you of all strength. A wish to prove that you need nothing, that you have no human hungers, which turns on itself and becomes a searing need for the hunger itself. It is an attempt to find an identity but ultimately strips you of any sense of yourself, save the sorry identity of "sick." It is a protest against cultural stereotypes of women that in the end makes you seem the weakest, the most needy and neurotic of all women. It is the thing you believe is keeping you safe, alive, contained—and in the end, of course, you find it's doing quite the opposite. (1999, 6)

The very ambiguity of people's experiences is thus not written away in this book, but brought to the forefront of relatedness. Abjection is premised on "ambiguity," a term I embrace, as it allows the ethnography to understand the complexities of anorexia while acknowledging the impossibility of explaining it completely. Thus my argument does not replace one rationalist explanation with another, for abjection and relatedness create interconnected spaces of transformation, ambiguity, and intersubjectivity rather than order, stasis, and predictability.

Future Directions

We know that anorexia and other eating disorders are a significant public health issue. In the United States, eating disorders affect more than five million people and are associated with "serious medical and psychiatric comorbidity" (Becker 2004b, 433). Anorexia can be devastating to everyone involved and can ruin lives and families. So how can this research help those with anorexia, families and friends, and those who treat them? It can help on a number of levels.

The first relates to how the knowledge presented in this book sits with current treatment programs/modalities. Clinicians know that anorexia is difficult to treat and that resistance to treatment is common (see also Fairburn and Harrison 2003). As I noted earlier in this book, there are a variety of treatment options available (from outpatient to inpatient to community programs), and they vary from country to country. Gremillion notes a swing back to inpatient programs in the United States, which demonstrates a tertiary (or end-stage) approach to those who need immediate clinical care. While she argues that programs have changed considerably in the last decade, she finds that "many practitioners today idealize programs like the one I studied [long-term inpatient hospitalization] and strive (or wish) to emulate its practices and principles as much as possible. Also, the centerpiece of most 'pared down' hospital programs remains, not surprisingly, weight gain through behavior modification. In fact, some hospital programs are now narrowing to this focus" (2003, 11).

Others argue that the future of treating anorexia lies in the new science of genomics, molecular pharmacology, and traditional clinical efforts (Strober 2005). In all these approaches to anorexia, the focus is primarily on biological needs and psychological changes, with the cultural context of anorexia receiving, at best, what Lee (2004) refers to as "lip service."

Yet what if we were to really unpack the place of culture in anorexia, beyond the standard culture-bound syndrome or what Lester (2007) refers to as the acculturation position? If we start to understand anorexia as an issue primarily concerned with local idioms of relatedness and abjection, then a broader conceptualization can occur. Anorexia, as the people in this study repeatedly argued, is not solely concerned with food and weight but is fundamentally concerned with issues of relatedness: of relationships with oneself, people, and objects in the world. Anorexia allowed participants to reformulate these relationships. Through a range of cleansing and ritualized practices, anorexia offers a way of managing abject relations, while simultaneously providing new and powerful forms of relatedness.

It is when we take this broader approach that we can see how experiences and treatments don't match up. Experiences are concerned with the wider net of relatedness (of displacement, connection, desire, and power), and treatment with narrow ideas coalescing around individual psychopathology (such as control, autonomy, and separation of mind and body). O'Connor and van Esterik (2008), in their call to demedicalize anorexia, suggest that traditional clinical hospital programs continue to decontextualize people with anorexia, and to reproduce this isolation via long-stay single-bed programs, cutting people off from the myriad of social contexts and relations around which food and bodies coalesce. Other work has also begun to highlight this counterproductive effect of treatment; in the reproduction of gendered family roles in the therapeutic team (Gremillion 2002, 2003; Moulding 2006), assumptions of normative female sexuality (Lester 2000), and the reproduction of anorexic spaces and practices (Warin 2005). Given these discrepancies and the unwitting reproduction of particular relationships, it is not surprising that institutional treatment has not been successful.

This mismatch between therapeutic interventions and what people with anorexia say about their experiences is even more pronounced when we look at the disorder across radically different cultural settings. Lester's comparative ethnographic work between Mexican and U.S. eating-disorder treatment centers highlights the frustration that clinicians in Mexico have with the dominant U.S. treatment models of individualism and autonomy. Clinicians in Mexico describe a mismatch between the theories and treatment strategies in which they have been trained (based on U.S. and European approaches) and what they encounter on the ground (Lester 2007, 377). The idea that treatment models should work toward reascribing values of independence and release from overinvolved mothers is anathema to "traditional Mexican values." This, Lester argues, is "out of synch with a [Mexican] cultural reality" in which people strive to become socially embedded and take an active, responsible role within a broader system of relationships (378). It is precisely this attention to social relatedness (rather than pathologizing forms of relating) that this book wants to underscore and bring to the fore in dominant models of understanding and treating anorexia.

The desire that coalesces around anorexia adds an ambiguity that defies the rational progress of clinical interventions. People in this research often spoke about their desire to be better anorexics in order to embody a sense of distinction and to belong. In a study of "pro-ana" Web sites, Giles argues that the pro-ana online community "affords a style of interaction that would be highly unlikely in the off-line, or pre-internet environment" (2006, 475). But this book clearly shows how this identity work of insiders/outsiders and the fierce contestation of identities' heroic moral subjectivities are absolutely central to the everyday practices of anorexia (see also Rich 2006; Gooldin 2008). It is this development of shared practices and knowledge coupled with gendered, moral virtues of personhood that needs to be considered in treatment paths. Again, in this desire to belong and embody the power of anorexia, healing, recovery and cure is anathema to the anorexic experience.

While Gremillion is correct in noting that most options for seriously ill people involve inpatient care, not all programs operate on a traditional model. One hospital in which I conducted fieldwork had ten different programs for people with eating disorders, the majority of which were outpatient based (only four inpatient beds were reserved for acute patients) (Warin 2005). Several features of this program distinguished it from the hospital programs in their reproduction of anorexic practices. First, Lane Cove was a community residential program located in a large three-story heritage home in the suburbs of Vancouver. Residents participated in a community, and this location changed the very nature of their identity (as they were not circumscribed by institutional walls, they did not consider themselves to be patients) and their recovery process.

The relationships between food and relatedness were central to this program, and people learned skills that would enable them to engage in social relationships when they left the program. These included sharing the preparation of food and cooking in the house kitchen, inviting friends and family members to share meals on certain nights, grocery shopping, participating in the day-to-day running of the house, and eating out. This service could be accessed only by those who had physically and emotionally prepared for a four-month stay through another supported program (which included reaching target weight prior to entering the program to circumvent competition between residents). The location of this treatment program unsettled and shifted the spatial relations of institutionalized power. Moreover, therapeutic spaces that supported the practices of anorexia (such as isolation in single bedrooms and eating alone) were challenged in an environment that focused on the fundamental relationships between sociality and food. As in Lester's account of Mexican treatments for anorexia, the goal for this program involved "a radical reformulation of a patient's understanding of herself, and more precisely, a reformulation of her self-in-relationship and the management of emotionality in relationships with others" (2007, 379–380). It is this emphasis on social relatedness and how one positions oneself in social relationships that needs to be incorporated into therapeutic environments.

Katzman and Lee (1997) have been suggesting for some time now that a shift in clinical interventions toward contextual variables may be useful. They suggest, for example, that "thinking about eating disorders as a problem of disconnection, transition, and oppression, rather than dieting, weight and fat phobia" would be beneficial to women with eating disorders who dwell "in a psychological diaspora" (Katzman and Lee 1997, 392). Certainly the cross-cultural work in populations undergoing rapid transition in the form of "migration, modernization, urbanization, and other economic, social and cultural changes" highlights the increased risk of eating disorders for young women (Becker 2004b, 433). This call to examine culture in the development of anorexia does not negate the potential of other equally important research agendas (such as neurobiology or epidemiological data) but calls for raising the value of an interpretive approach in a field that is currently dominated by clinical discourse.

Of course, this would mean arguing for certain methodological approaches that are often overlooked as they do not conform to assumptions about objectivity, fact, and replicability. As Barrett (1996) argues in his meticulous examination of the social definition of schizophrenia, the purpose of positivist science is to produce a form of knowledge that is isolated from its context. Converting data into variables allows standardization, population comparisons, and correlations. In contrast, ethnographic inquiry brings the context into focus. It demonstrates the importance of careful attention to a person's habitus, and the daily practices and details of everyday life. This context includes both the field of diagnosis and the phenomenological shaping of illness experience. This detailed context can help us to reimagine how we might help people with anorexia, and how those with a diagnosis might begin to conceptualize what help they might need.

There are growing calls to think about new approaches to anorexia. Pike and Borovoy (2004) suggest that to study eating disorders without a discussion of culture is tantamount to watching actors on a stage with no set design. Lee (2004, 617) similarly argues that "engaging culture is an overdue task for eating disorder research." In examining the social life of anorexia across three cultural sites, my work points to the ways in which women use food and their bodies to negotiate the complexity and ambiguity of social relatedness. I do not suggest that there is a single or universal experience of anorexia, or that other biocultural factors are not implicated. I do, however, suggest that experiences of anorexia are drawn from a common set of cultural practices relating to how women understand their bodies and everyday, gendered practices around relatedness. It is these local worlds of bodies, desire, and disgust that lead us to wider issues of belonging, connection, and disconnection, all of which resonate with comparative ethnographic work on eating disorders.

NOTES

CHAPTER 1 INTRODUCTION

1. Pseudonyms have been used for participants throughout this book except in the case of one woman who requested that her name not be changed, as she felt that this was an important part of her recovery and of who she is.
2. Marilyn Strathern acknowledges Schneider as "the anthropological father" of *After Nature*, "since it is both with and against his ideas on kinship that [her book] is written" (1992, xviii).
3. The average age was twenty-eight, belying the stereotype of people with anorexia as in their early teens.
4. Lester (2000) provides an illuminating account of how sexual abstinence in anorexia is clinically constructed in relation to normative constructions of sexuality and femininity.
5. As Jenkins and Barrett note in their edited volume on schizophrenia, a Janus-faced approach is necessary in such an effort, as one must work with the clinical category as it is currently defined (schizophrenia or anorexia) and at the same time subject it to cultural critique (2004, 4–5). Moreover, this book does not subscribe to the common assumption that anorexia exists independently of bulimia or eating disorders not otherwise specified (categorized by the acronym EDNOS). The American Psychiatric Association's Work Group on Eating Disorders reflects the intermingling of eating disorders when it describes anorexia nervosa as "a continuum between anorexia and bulimia, [with] many patients demonstrating a mixture of both anorexic and bulimic behaviors" (2000, 19).
6. I found an implicit assumption among some female audience members at seminar presentations of this research that simply being a woman made one an authority and gave one authenticity for all women's experience. Tsing, citing Strathern's arguments in *The Gender of the Gift* (1988), warns against the easy assumptions "that women everywhere are the same; that women's speech reveals a 'woman's point of view'; that women always speak from the gender identity of 'woman.' Strathern stresses the necessity of investigating the forms of power and discourse framed by the exclusions and oppositions of gender; these become the starting point for discussing both the 'femaleness' and the 'agency' of women's agency" (Tsing 1993, 33).
7. Bray lists the many significations of anorexia, concluding that "this taxonomy demonstrates that the body of the woman who practices eating disorders presents a coding problem. As the 'dark continent of femininity,' the territory of the anorexic body has been colonised by a motley group of discourses contesting the truth of anorexic lack" (1996, 413–414).

8. Popular and medical literature is replete with examples of "anorexics" looking in the mirror and seeing an imaginary body that belies their emaciated form. Similarly, when people with anorexia are asked to draw their physical body, they are said to exaggerate their size. The current emphasis on thinness is not in accordance with people's own representations or renderings.
9. People with HIV/AIDS, though, are similarly represented in a process of death. What fascinates and horrifies for both anorexia and AIDS is the closeness of death in the prime of life.
10. One psychiatrist asked me if I was aware that it was very fashionable to study anorexia, pointing to the double exoticism of anorexia and psychiatry. Anorexia is fashionable in the sense that it is more spectacular than other eating disorders. The media privileges anorexia through glamorization and fetishization of this disorder, as exemplified by the Australian weeknight television program (*A Current Affair*) that followed a young woman's experience of anorexia and treatment over three years. Not once during my fieldwork did I see the same program hosting a special on bulimia or compulsive eating. These disorders do not offer the horror or spectacle of the wasted anorexic body and are therefore not considered high rating. Gordon (a professor of psychology and practicing clinical psychologist), in his book *Eating Disorders: Anatomy of a Social Epidemic*, highlights the way in which the media has had a hand in popularizing some psychiatric disorders: "During the late 1970s and early 1980s, anorexia nervosa was widely publicized, glamorized, and to some extent romanticized. Language such as 'disorder of the 80s' reflects the fact that in the era of modern media, diseases, and particularly psychiatric disorders, can easily become fashionable and popularized, and this was indeed the case for anorexia nervosa" (2000, 3). Malson (a lecturer in psychology) similarly notes: "The high profile of 'anorexia nervosa' in both the popular and academic press suggests a cultural fascination with eating disorders" (1998, 5).
11. A brief review of Malson's recent book *The Thin Woman* (1998), for example, illustrates this alliance with Foucault's concept of discourse; seven of the eight chapter titles include a derivative of the word "discourse": discoursing, discursive, or discursive productions.
12. Eckermann, among others, similarly criticizes feminist writers such as Orbach and Lawrence who have embraced Bruch's (1978) leanings "towards a causal model of the media as directly responsible for all social ills, and anorexia in particular as a falling out from experiencing too much representation" (Eckermann 1994, 92).
13. Grosz makes a similar point concerning the close analogy between the body and the text (1994, 117). She also suggests that while Bordo's discussion of anorexia in terms of a psychology of self-control is extremely useful, it risks duplicating the mind/body dualism and taking the body as a kind of natural bedrock to which psychological and sociological analyses may be added as cultural overlays (145).
14. Foucault recognized the overemphasis on "techniques of domination" in institutions and shifted his later work into "technologies of the self" (Foucault 1980, cited in Miller 1993, 321–322; see also Foucault 1990). The overemphasis on hegemonic power is demonstrated in Barrett's ethnography, where he explicitly links Gramsci's concept of hegemonic power to Foucault's more diffuse and uncentralized power (Barrett 1996, 73; see also Frankenberg 1988).
15. In "The Other Question: Difference, Discrimination, and the Discourse of Colonialism," Homi Bhabha similarly argues that some theorists overemphasize the

hegemony of colonial discourse, such as, in his view, Edward Said: "There is always, in Said, the suggestion that colonial power and discourse [are] possessed entirely by the colonizer" (1990, 77).

16. Glick (1967) notes that "access to power and the ability to employ it on behalf of the sufferer is universally required if one is to be considered a healer" (cited in Good 1994, 60).

17. Eckermann suggests that Foucauldian formulations of power are explicitly tied to a particular construction of selfhood. As an example, she cites the work of Giddens (1991), who argues that anorexia is a search for selfhood, the production of a coherent, consonant, and unitary self. Giddens's reliance on the discursive construction of the self, Eckermann argues, does not allow for multiple, embodied, and contradictory forms of power and identity (1994, 89–90).

18. Probyn has experienced firsthand the ways in which a discursive construction of identity can be limiting. In delivering a conference paper, she stated in a passing comment: "I became anorexic." These three words caused consternation in the audience, with one person saying that "this personal mode of enunciation made him nervous" (1993, 12). Following publication of the paper, Probyn was further rebuked on the one hand for absenting her own anorexic body from the text (Szekely 1988, 10) and on the other hand for writing her own "postmodern ethnography" (Frank 1990, 146–148). What perplexed Probyn was that all three (different) reactions assumed an essential and static truth of her personal identity, "that I was telling, or wanting to tell, the truth, in this case about the essence of my being" (Probyn 1993, 12). Moreover, these reactions suggest a divide between objectivist and subjective knowledges and articulations, between writing too much and too little of herself into the work.

19. As I was doing the research for this book, the lead singer (Daniel Johns) of a three-piece Australian band, Silverchair, wrote "Ana's Song," about his recent experiences of anorexia. One participant developed a close connection with this song, using her hospital free time to catch a bus to the local shopping center to buy the new CD (and showing me the album cover and reading the lyrics out to me), pinning posters of the singer and band on the walls of her single hospital room, and even writing to Daniel Johns from her hospital bed to convey empathy. Very early on in our relationship, this young woman excitedly played this song to me, as she considered that the music and poetic lyrics conveyed what she said was unspeakable about her own experiences.

20. Parkin, Gell, Moeran, and Weiner debated precisely this issue: "whether language calls into being the cultural worlds in which people live, or whether these worlds are given form and meaning by virtue of cognitive engagement that preceded language" (Ingold 1992, 1). I side with the two debaters who argue that language is not the essence of culture, for "culture consists of concepts rather than verbally constituted meanings, and that these concepts are established in the course of a direct, practical involvement with other persons and things in one's surroundings, an involvement which need not (and for small children does not) entail fully fledged verbal discourse; . . . [it] includes all kinds of everyday non-linguistic practices as well." One conclusion of this debate was that any attempt to draw language and culture apart would lead to the "absurdities of culturally decontextualized language and linguistically decontextualized culture" (2).

21. A criticism leveled at phenomenology is that in describing what comes into view within immediate experience (or even in thinking about what comes into view),

one necessarily draws on language, and therefore one is not studying experience at all, but the representation of experience through language. Yet phenomenology, in providing "detailed descriptions of how people immediately experience space, time and the world in which they live," arrives not at presuppositionless description of phenomena, but at a reinterpretation—as new meaning, or renewed meaning (Jackson 1996, 12).

22. Bourdieu takes issue with phenomenology for what he sees as its failure to appreciate that agents classify and construct their understandings of the social world from particular positions in a hierarchically structured social space (Swartz 1997, 57; Bourdieu 1990, 26–27). Yet I would argue that his theory of habitus draws from a mixture of phenomenology and structuralism. Jackson makes exactly my point: "Despite his caveats and cavils, Bourdieu's emphasis on mundane strategizing, practical taxonomies, bodily habits, social usages, and agency makes his notion of *habitus* directly comparable to the notion of lifeworld" (1996, 20). For a fuller investigation of Bourdieu's relationship to phenomenology, see Throop and Murphy 2002.

23. Even the assumption that anorexia is primarily linked to food is challenged in this book. Food, in its commonsense meaning of nutrition, pleasure, and sustenance, is disrupted by experiences of these substances as invading, polluting, or even poisoning.

24. Certainly there has been what Geurts refers to as a "renaissance in the senses" (2002, 13) in such ethnographic works as Dennis 2007; Desjarlais 2003; Howes 1991, 2003; Roseman 1991; Seremetakis 1994; and Stoller 1989, 1997. Medical anthropologists have only recently begun to examine somatic symptoms and qualia, as evidenced by the recent call to develop a medical anthropology of the senses (Hinton, Howes, and Kirmayer 2008; Nichter 2008).

CHAPTER 2 STEERING A COURSE BETWEEN FIELDS

1. Barrett notes that "multidisciplinary teams arose within mental health services during the 1960s as part of a widespread expansion and reform of psychiatric hospitals throughout the developed world" (1996, 74).

2. In *Fluid Signs*, Daniel discusses the central role of movement (both physical and intellectual) in anthropological methodology: "A cultural account is by definition an interpretive account, and as an interpretive account it must be capable of conveying information even as a metaphor does. Interpretation entails a movement, a movement that brings the interpretive subject and the interpretive object together in partial coalescence" (1984, 52).

3. I could have placed an advertisement for participants in a local paper—Garrett (1998) recruited participants for her study of spiritual narratives of recovery from anorexia in the *Sydney Morning Herald*)—but I wanted access to hospitals as well.

4. This democratic process of group members having the final decision as to my entry reflected the measure of control that was purposively afforded to residents. Lane Cove was very much the residents' space, and unlike a hospital setting, they felt they had control and responsibility for what happened under its roof.

5. Malson and Ussher note that the weight of the interviewer in their study was central to relationships: "As a thin woman of a similar age to many of the interviewees,

the interviewer's own subject positions may have been significant in diminishing the power differential between researcher and the researched since there was a sharing of some subject positions and experiences. The (partial) sharing of discourses, subject positions and experiences between interviewer and interviewees will have had some effect on the dynamics of the interview process and, thereby, on the ways in which the interviewees articulated their ideas and experiences" (1996, 509).

6. I do not share the view put forward in Lévi-Strauss 1973, 1981; in Bourdieu 1990; or by Geertz that suggests that all forms of phenomenology are "privacy theories of meaning" (1973, 12) or simply a philosophy of the self. Such an understanding of social phenomenology is in my view limited and flawed. Jackson, citing Merleau-Ponty, argues that "praxis is seldom a matter of individuals acting alone. It is a mode of shared endeavor as well as conflict, of mutual adjustment as well as violence. Subjectivity is in effect a matter of intersubjectivity and experience is interexperience" (Merleau-Ponty 1973, 56, cited in Jackson 1996, 26).
7. Burrill Crohn was a U.S. gastroenterologist (1884–1983); Thomas Addison (1793–1860) and James Parkinson (1755–1824) were English physicians (Stedman 1995).
8. From a biological point of view, metabolic and hormonal disturbances were called into question when trying to explicate anorexia. Psychoanalysts contended that food refusal was a defense against oral impregnation (see also Freud 1958, 268); behavioralists argued that people with anorexia needed conditioned hospital environments where weight gain could be monitored and positively reinforced (see also Gremillion 1992, 62). From a psychodynamic point of view, people with anorexia are represented as being afraid of sexual maturation and female growth, preferring to live a "childish, asexual life" (Vandereycken and van Deth 1994, 3). Others viewed anorexia as a sign of disturbed structures and interactions within the family. There are also many different ways of treating anorexia within these models.
9. I thank the late Dr. Kingsley Garbett for sharing and discussing his opinions on these differences with me.
10. The terms "client" and "patient" circulate in different contexts; each has a clear political agenda (see also Taussig 1980).
11. This positionality of "I know because I've been there" is, as Moore notes, "particularly troublesome when linked to grounds of authority." What worries Moore is the way in which "experience is reduced to its linguistic and cognitive elements, . . . encouraging a view of experience which sees it as ontological, singular and fixed" (1994, 2).
12. The American Psychiatric Association reflects this experiential dimension of eating disorders and describes anorexia nervosa as "a continuum between anorexia and bulimia, [with] many patients demonstrating a mixture of both anorexic and bulimic behaviors" (2000, 19).
13. The term "narrative" has currency within medicine and anthropology, as epitomized by the development of the term "illness narratives" by Arthur Kleinman (1988), himself a psychiatrist and anthropologist. Narrative, though, is understood differently in each field and cannot be transferred or taken unproblematically across fields. Anthropologists have taken on board, criticized, and extended the usefulness of narrative in fieldwork (see Rapport 2000, which focuses solely on the transcription of words; J. Weiner 1995, which disparages narratives as "feeble

anthropology"; and Good 1994, which foregrounds experience as prior to narrative). The sticking point in these different uses of "narrative" centers on the literary constructions of the term and the fields (or lack of) in which they are constituted. Illness narratives, according to Kleinman, are like literary texts, consisting of "content, structure, rhetorical devices, plot, and story line" (1988, 233). In critiquing this model, Saris (1995) and Lucas (1999), for example, point to the "symbolic violence" embedded in the collection and interpretation of illness narratives, the institutional contexts in which they are framed, and the relationship between agency, meaning, and power. Moreover, Lucas suggests that the indeterminate ways of "telling a story" are not simply about words, they are also about gestures, images, silences, and erasures. He suggests that the ways in which *agency* is manifest as storytelling, of how it is constituted (and not just mediated) by an institutional field, is a more interesting question (1999, 12).

14. Similarly, Lester's (2007) critique of the acculturation hypothesis using a cross-cultural comparison between the treatment of anorexia in Mexico and the United States demonstrates that the clinical category or reality of this disorder is contentious.

CHAPTER 3 KNOWING THROUGH THE BODY

1. "Commensality" traditionally means "those that gather around a table to share food" (Visser 1992, 83). My use of "commensality" extends to a much wider habitus: the embodied rules of etiquette, hygiene, and spaces of commensality; and the exchange of sensory memories, emotions, substances, and material objects that are embedded in shared histories (Seremetakis 1994).
2. Many people with illnesses or conditions that are diet related (such as diabetes, high cholesterol, or allergies) are all too aware of the readiness-to-hand of food. Illness and health is one area where the taken-for-granted nature of one's embodiment is thrown into relief.
3. Connecting feelings to eating is an integral part of cognitive behavioral therapy, a popular form of treatment for eating disorders.
4. The practice of eating itself could not be taken for granted, as participants had different types of eating: binge eating, for example, was characterized as hurriedly eating large amounts of food and was viewed as dangerous (in terms of desire) and redolent with emotion.
5. Wafer notes the romantic imaginings of the field: "'The field' has various resonances; it evokes, simultaneously, peripherality and nature (since fields are in the country), and 'the real world' (as distinct from the library or the laboratory). It is thus a romantic notion, because it suggests the possibility of an alternative to the centralization, artifice, and 'unreality' of contemporary intellectual life" (1996, 260).
6. Over time, the strangeness of the field dissipates and it becomes familiar. Kondo momentarily gazed at the reflection of a typical Japanese housewife in a shop window before realizing that she had "caught a glimpse of nothing less than [her] own reflection" (1986, 74). Coming home or out of the field, rather than being a return to familiarity, can be a profoundly disorientating and disturbing experience, as Desjarlais notes: "When I left Nepal, I could not shake off the sensibilities that helped me get about, and found, when I tried to speak with

friends or buy a pair of sneakers, that I had lost the knack of being American" (Desjarlais 1992, 251).

7. While Edwards does discuss and defend her choice of ethnographic locale in her homeland of Britain, she also suggests, and I agree with her, that the time has come for debates about anthropology at home to move on: "There is something unhelpful, it seems to me, in perpetuating the notion that there is an anthropology at home, which then requires, as its counterpart, an anthropology elsewhere. We need to focus attention instead on the way in which certain items of information come to be of anthropological interest—to tease out some of our reasons for homing-in on certain things and not others—and this requires more than a methodological reflexivity" (2000, 11).
8. There were also times when I ate communally with the staff of eating-disorder units.
9. Female staff in one eating-disorder unit discussed the importance of their size in terms of establishing and maintaining relationships with clients. A social worker recounted that patients had told her, "I feel I can trust you because you're slim." Participants similarly told me that they could not trust staff who were overweight. One young woman exclaimed, "How am I meant to trust Jenny [a dietitian] when she's overweight herself? She obviously has her own issues with food" (see also Katzman 1993).
10. Hastrup makes a point similar to Jackson's: "While we cannot, obviously, experience the world from the perspective of others, we can still share their social experience. In fact, there is no social experience that is not shared; . . . ethnography is based in a social experience that is shared by the ethnographer and 'her people'" (1995, 51).
11. Abu-Lughod reflects on the ways in which different but common experiences bring women together (1995, 347). "A Tale of Two Pregnancies" is concerned with Abu-Lughod's experience of being pregnant and the lives of the women with whom she spent her fieldwork time in the Western Desert of Egypt.
12. Hornbacher captures the uncanny presence of death in her own experiences of anorexia: "Death is at your shoulder, death is your shadow, your scent, your waking and dreaming companion" (1999, 125).
13. In discussing her own embodied acculturation of Malay symbolism, Laderman writes: "Anthropologists use their own bodies and minds as primary tools for the investigation of cultures. They participate as deeply as possible in the lives of those they study, at the same time maintaining sufficient distance to observe the workings of culture. They become insider-outsiders" (1994, 192).

CHAPTER 4 THE COMPLEXITIES OF BEING ANOREXIC

1. In expanding her notion of "outside," Probyn also draws on Foucault's concept of heterotopia, for it "provides an analytic space in which to consider forms of belonging outside the divisiveness of categorizing" (Probyn 1996, 10). Heterotopia juxtaposes in one real place several different spaces, "several sites that are in themselves incompatible or foreign to one another" (Foucault, cited in Soja 1995, 15). As Edward Soja puts it, these are "places where many spaces converge and become entangled" (1995, 15). As both inside and outside, heterotopic spaces are inextricably double, and foreground the changing configurations of social relations. In this formulation,

hospital spaces were sites of heterotopia, where the possibilities of being anorexic and not being anorexic were played out.

2. I recognize that this mapping could be an effect of psychiatric or therapeutic intervention, where patients are encouraged to tell their stories and rationalize them. Fiona Place, in her autobiographical story *Cardboard Lives*, suggests: "Life, for people who have been using anorexic eyes/metaphors long term, has often become only the description of the symptoms of their illness, and possibly of numerous admissions and discharges over the years or experiences of other methods of treatment. They so often reach the stage whereby they give their life history as a psychiatric history, using solely the associated jargon and therefore experiencing it as such" (1989, 257).

3. Bettina said that over the years she had spent "thousands of dollars" on skin care products, treatments, and minor cosmetic surgery in her quest to achieve this perfection.

4. Maddy's productive desire for other women came after she had "recovered" from anorexia. Until then, she spent a number of years confused and angry at her male partner's sexual liaisons with men as he continued a sexual relationship with her. His behavior led her to question her desirability, to wonder whether he had simply been attracted to her because, as she recounted, "I'm a bit of a tomboy and I don't have a curvy figure or big breasts."

5. Holden (1991) has noted the higher than average rates of adoption among patients admitted for eating disorders to the Maudsley psychiatric hospital in London compared to the general population.

6. Alienation is undeniably disempowering, as Peters writes: "Most A.N's [anorexics] claim feeling powerless . . . This can be linked to feeling alienated from the body. Berger and Luckman (1966) explain that most humans hover in the balance between being and having a body. All my informants claimed they felt marginal, alienated and powerless. They associated this to their experience of their bodies. This feeling of alienation extends beyond the family; its locus is cultural and it affects all women in varying degrees" (1987). While participants in my research recounted similar feelings of displacement, they also spoke at length about the incredible power that alienation from their bodies gave them. Exclusion and alienation can create their own power.

7. Several participants displayed a hatred for their own flesh by cutting or burning their skin, with the aim of allowing the emotive properties contained in their blood to drain away.

8. Other writers have commented on the desire of those with anorexia to become androgynous or malelike (see Malson 1998, 114). Bruch reports "that many anorexics, when children, dreamt and fantasized about growing up to be boys" (1979, cited in Bordo 1988, 102). Bordo notes a woman who commented: "If only [I] could stay thin, . . . I would never have to deal with having a woman's body; like Peter Pan I could stay a child forever." The choice of Peter Pan, Bordo suggests, is telling: "what she means is, stay a *boy* forever" (102).

9. It is interesting—and I have Margie Ripper to thank for pointing this out to me—that Robert does not think of sexuality as his desire but as being desired (or not), that is, attractive or unattractive to others.

10. Hornbacher (1999, 106) also describes the connections that occurred in treatment settings: "at first there is a religious fervour, a cultist sort of behavior, a pact. I made a pact with a tall, thin girl who offered to help me lose weight."
11. See Crow, Keel, and Kendall 1998 for a review of the literature regarding eating disorders and insulin-dependent diabetes.
12. Bray and Colebrook note that Deleuze in *Dialogues* "refers to anorexia as a phenomenon that has been subjected to misinterpretation precisely to the degree that it has been organized according to a theory of lack" (Deleuze 1987, 90, 111, cited in Bray and Colebrook 1998, 63).
13. Rich (2006) similarly notes how inpatients "skank" and "tank" their food in an effort to avoid food and share "anorexic practices."
14. This description of "pulling tricks" could be applied to the tactics of shoplifting, a phenomenon that has been reported as significantly higher among women with eating disorders (Baum and Goldner 1995; Goldner et al. 2000). Goldner and colleagues suggest that the association of shoplifting with eating-disorder severity may be due to "mental dysfunction associated with the starvation and metabolic compromise that often accompany severe eating disorders." I would argue that there are other important dimensions at play, such as the effects of cheating a powerful capitalist-driven system. At ward rounds during my fieldwork there were several references to women who had been caught stealing laxatives and were awaiting criminal prosecution. Goldner and colleagues similarly note that the women in their study who were using laxatives reported stealing them, suggesting that this was "motivated in part by a desire to maintain the secrecy of their purgative methods" (474).
15. In her book *The Secret Language of Eating Disorders*, Claude-Pierre similarly notes the excuses and "tricks" that patients use to avoid foods: "'I can't eat this bread because it bothers my gums.' 'I'm diabetic, so I can't have sugar.' 'I'm lactose intolerant, so I can't have milk.' 'I'm hypoglycemic, so I can't have fat'" (1997, 102).
16. Gooldin (2008) also notes how participants in her study related feelings of hunger to a sense of achievement, in which "being anorexic" is constructed as a "heroic project." Richard O'Connor and Penny van Esterik (2008) similarly comment on the strong sense of achievement and pride that women with anorexia attach to their own ascetic lives and identity.
17. Barth's study of the secretive men's initiation cult among the New Guinea Baktaman describes the accumulation of status that comes with the learning of more in-depth knowledge. The ascending stages of concealment and revelation each carries greater status: "Each level is organized so as to obscure the next level; . . . he [the initiate] realizes the existence of veil behind veil" (1975, 219–220).
18. In explaining *la perruque*, de Certeau uses military language, such as "enemies," "battle lines," "soldiers," and "struggles") as a metaphor. The same military language is utilized by those with anorexia.
19. One therapist told me how a former group of residents at Lane Cove had developed "underground behaviors." Collectively they had agreed not to use oil when cooking the evening meals and to hide this decision (and practice) from staff. Another participant recalled how she had once co-opted a patient on the psychiatric ward who did not have an eating disorder to buy laxatives for her at the hospital shop.
20. Once diagnosed with "the wasting disease," people felt that they had to uphold the stereotype of being thin or be deemed a fraud. Maintaining the stereotype people told me, made it difficult to recover.

21. Unlike Harris (1989) and Carrithers, Collins, and Lukes (1985), I do not understand the concepts of self and other to be in opposition. The assumed dichotomy of self/person, which is premised on a biological/social ontology, suggests that the self is "a locus of individual [and universal] experience, through its counterposition to the person as a being formed within the moral framework of society and its relationships" (Ingold 1991, 365). As Ingold argues, people do not come into being as selves prior to their entry into social relationships: "selves become, and they do so within a matrix of relations with others" (367).
22. I often asked those participants who had personified anorexia what gender it was. It was sometimes female and sometimes male.
23. Bemis-Vitousek similarly describes "the honeymoon phase of eating disorders" as like "the romance of a new marriage" (1997, 9).

CHAPTER 5 ABJECT RELATIONS WITH FOOD

1. Weber's *The Protestant Ethic and the Spirit of Capitalism* (1930) also clearly made this connection between Christian asceticism and the rise of science.
2. While I agree with this argument, it is located within a particular historical (and cultural) period. Mennell (1991, 138) notes that medicalization had little impact on the dietary regimes of those who were not ill prior to the "modern era"; along the lines of Norbert Elias, he argues that it was "the progressive move towards the 'civilizing' of appetite, with its emphasis on refinement, delicacy and self-control as a sign of courtly manners, rather than explicitly medical reasons that began to change dietary habits in Europe in the sixteenth and seventeenth centuries" (Mennell 1985, cited in Lupton 1996, 68). And of course, earlier still were the Hippocratic injunctions concerning personal hygiene and a balanced diet for good health. For a comprehensive overview of attitudes to food in late antiquity see Grimm 1996.
3. Coveney (1998, 1999, 2000/2006) uses Foucault's insights to characterize the ways in which people, populations, the public, and individuals are disciplined by nutritional discourses.
4. Austin (1999) argues that public health promoters have unwittingly served to fuel "obsessive concerns with food, fat and diet" (1999, 263).
5. Santich (1995) describes the way "nutrition encourages a 'good'/'bad' dichotomy by producing a food hierarchy based on what is considered nutritious" (1995, 146, cited in Coveney 2000, 28).
6. This dietary message is manifest in the brand-name advertising of foods such as Lean Cuisine, Lite, and Healthy Choice.
7. Eckermann claims that "research continues to show a relationship between 'eating disorders' and religious affiliation" (1994, 94). One such study reported a strong correlation between Catholic and Jewish women and eating disorders (Sykes, Gross, and Subishin 1986).
8. Malson notes the variations in percentage weight loss considered necessary for diagnosis: "Whereas *IDC-10* (WHO 1992) and *DSM-III-R* (APA 1987) [and *DSM-IV* (APA 1994)] state that weight loss (or lack of expected weight gain) should be at least 15 per cent, *DSM-III* (APA 1980) states 25 per cent and others (for example, Meskey 1980) state 20 per cent. Precisely how much weight a woman has to lose before she

is pathologized seems to vary, and to some extent the decision is arbitrary" (Malson 1998, 3).

9. Although fear of fat or fat phobia is central to the Western diagnosis of anorexia, a number of commentators argue that it is not a universal feature (see also Lee 2001). In reviewing the literature, Katzman and Lee (1997) highlight studies that do not support the taken-for-granted diagnostic assumption of fat phobia. Lee, Ho, and Hsu 1993, for example, reports no fear of becoming fat amongst anorexic patients in Hong Kong. Kok and Tian 1994 similarly reports no fat phobia in large-scale surveys among those with anorexia in Singapore.

10. One exception is MacSween, who investigated what foods women with anorexia ate, why they chose particular foods, which were their favorite foods, and what they would never eat. She concluded that food in anorexia is separated into two distinct categories: food as safe (low calorie and nonfattening) and as dangerous (pleasurable and fattening). "Food that gives pleasure is dangerous food; the aim is to eliminate the pleasure, and eventually the food itself" (1993, 215). While MacSween introduces Douglas's (1984) concept of "matter out of place," it is ritual rather than pollution that she focuses on: "For the anorexic woman all eating is dangerous and transitional, and ritualization is an attempt to make it progressively safer by divesting it as far as possible of spontaneity and response to desire" (MacSween 1993, 207).

11. I am aware of excluding fluids in this discussion.

12. Succeeding citations of this source will appear in the text as page numbers in parentheses.

13. When I went to visit Rita with my baby daughter, she exclaimed how pleased she was that Freya was being breast-fed and had not yet been contaminated by food. In Rita's eyes, Freya thus was "pure."

14. In Shute's novel *Life-Size* (1992), there are similar equations of food with bodily waste products. In writing from her hospital bed about her experiences of anorexia, Josie described food as like excrement, mucous, and urine.

15. Two participants found the stickiness (rather than the caloric content) of jam and honey to be most problematic. Douglas, quoting Sartre from *Being and Nothingness* (1943), notes the horror and ambiguity of things which are sticky: "the viscous is a state half-way between solid and liquid . . . it is unstable . . . it attacks the boundary between myself and it; . . . to touch stickiness is to risk diluting myself into viscosity" (Douglas 1984, 38).

16. Counihan reproduces this metaphoric transposition of body to society in her brief analysis of eating disorders. She cites Douglas's argument in order to explain fasting: "Mary Douglas asserts that the 'human body is always treated as an image of society' and that the passage of food in and out of the body can stand for social boundaries and their transgression (1973, 70). Most important for our concerns here is her claim that 'bodily control is an expression of social control' (ibid). Western women's strong concern to control their food intake is a metaphor for their efforts to control their own bodies and destinies in a culture that makes self control a moral imperative" (1999, 99–100). Garrett similarly draws on Douglas's themes in her analysis of anorexia as a purity ritual. She argues that "the body" of anorexia is used as "a diagram of a social situation," as "a personal ritual that is an attempted solution to social problems." Moreover, while she critiques Kim Chernin's (1986) problematic distinction of nature/culture, she reproduces a number of dichotomies (of individual/society and nature/culture) in her own work. She characterizes

anorexia, for example, as "a ritual which represents rejection of life and connection with nature, . . . the fear of connection between the individual and the outer world" (1992, 14).

17. Jackson similarly critiques this representational bias in the anthropology of the body, using the disembodied nature of Douglas's work as example: "The human body [in these writings] is simply an object of understanding or an instrument of the rational mind, a kind of vehicle for the expression of a reified social rationality; . . . subjugation of the bodily to the semantic is empirically untenable; . . . meaning should not be reduced to a sign which, as it were, lies on a separate plane outside the immediate domain of the act" (1989, 122–123, cited in Csordas 1994, 10). In exploring bodily experiences, Jackson calls for evocation rather than representation, a task that should be phenomenological in nature (205–208).

18. Although desire is central to Kristeva's concept of abjection, it is linked to a psychoanalytic (Lacanian) legacy of negativity. This ethnography, however, clearly demonstrates the ways in which desire is experienced as both lack *and* productive force. I thank Melissa Iocco and Ingrid Hofmann for making this clear for me.

19. Kristeva's interest in the maternal, food, death, and the text are strikingly similar to Bakhtin's concept of grotesque. Kristeva wrote about Bakhtin's intertextuality and dialogism in her essay "Word, Dialogue, and Novel" (1966), a year after Bakhtin's *Rabelais and His World* was published. In that essay, and in *Powers of Horror*, Kristeva mentions Bakhtin's use of carnival only in passing. Her concept of abjection could be seen, as Vice states, "as a psychoanalytically inflected development of Bakhtin's grotesque. Even if the link between the two concepts is not that of Kristeva's debt to Bakhtin, Kristeva's model offers a different and more modern way of viewing the same phenomena Bakhtin discusses. Rather than contradicting Bakhtin's theory, hers can be seen as an extension of his" (1997, 163).

20. Malson notes in her study that some people could not even say the word "food"; one of her female interviewees said: "You'll find that I never say f-double-o-d—uh. There are certain words that are just taboo such as e-a-t-i-n-g as well. I wouldn't say that to save my life. . . . I look at these things as being poison and I don't want poison in my body and I want to be cleansed inside" (1998, 128).

21. Kristeva's reading of anthropology equates it and its "subjects" with "the primitive." She refers to "primitives" as people who have a lot in common with European children, poets, and psychotics. Moreover, as Tsing also notes: "*Powers of Horror* follows an insulting evolutionary track [a biologized scheme of pan-human development] from Africans and Indians to Judaism, Christianity, and, at last, to French poets. In addition, she assumes an epistemological dichotomy between European 'theory' and global 'empirical' variation in which, by definition, the Third World can never be a source of theoretical insight" (Tsing 1993, 180–181). Tsing continues to provide a powerful critique of Kristeva's singular and universalized treatment of gender, and of the ways in which she sees gender difference as prior to culture (the maternal is the ground from which all phallic culture emerges) (186).

22. It was not only foods that were hungered after, but also relationships and intimacy. Natalia had written in her diaries about "skin hunger," a term that she used to describe the strong desires that some people with eating disorders have to be touched.

23. In *The Forgetting of Air in Martin Heidegger* (1999), Irigaray critiques the metaphysical tradition that the work of Heidegger (and other philosophers) is founded upon—that is, the solid earth. She argues that there can be no presence, or Being, without air, yet its fluid, invisible, transparent nature renders it forgotten.

24. The two factors that aided the rise and fear of miasma were air and heat. In his history of odor and the French social imagination, Corbin notes that, before the advance in what was called pneumatic chemistry in 1750, air was thought to act as a passive carrier, transporting an accumulation of foreign particles (1996, 11–12). Air was believed to act on the living body in multiple ways: by simple contact with the skin or pulmonary membranes, by exchanges through the pores, and by direct ingestion. The temperature and humidity of air was central to its effects on the body. Participants often spoke of this combined fear of temperature and air with reference to cooking food. Barbecues were the worst offenders. The sound of sizzling fat and the smell of cooking meat turned people's stomachs, and many could not be in the vicinity of such smells for fear of inhaling the polluting vapors. The heat of cooking added potency to the food.

25. An Australian advertisement for a plastic food wrap (Clingfilm) depicts a male surgeon in an operating theatre (supposedly one of the most sterile environments) wrapping food in antibacterial wrap.

26. In reflecting on the ways in which her roommate takes all aspects of food for granted, Hornbacher describes her as having "no idea" about Hornbacher's own intense fears and desires surrounding butter: "The idea of buying butter in a store, the idea of touching butter without fear that the oils would seep through the skin of your fingers and make a little lipidy beeline for your butt, the idea of eating food that you knew, you knew had butter in it, of having butter in your possession that did not haunt your waking and sleeping hours, that did not wear a little invisible sign that only you saw: EAT ME, ALL OF ME. NOW" (1999, 265).

27. It is widely acknowledged that despite their abhorrence of food, people with anorexia often work in restaurants or catering industries. Those in my research who worked around food and prepared it for others explained that the proximity visually satiated their hunger. They simultaneously maintained a distance through the use of plastic gloves, tongs, or frequent hand washing.

28. In a Freudian analysis on Ndembu color symbolism, Turner suggests that "we" understand the basic color triad (black, white, and red) preconceptually in terms of universal human bodily and visceral experience. The three colors "stand for basic human experiences of the body (associated with gratification of libido, hunger, aggressive and excretory drives, and with fear, anxiety, and submissiveness)" (Turner 1970, 89–90 cited in Jackson 1998, 82–83). Such a universalized, decontextualized, and disembodied schema typifies (and renders problematic) psychoanalytical analysis, as my critique of Kristeva suggests. The importance of the color red is expanded in the next chapter in relation to a particular context of bodily fluids, gender, and sexuality.

CHAPTER 6 "ME AND MY DISGUSTING BODY"

1. The most recent diagnostic manual *DSM-IV* (American Psychiatric Association 1994) changes the word "abuse" to "misuse."

2. When participants arrived at one psychiatric ward, they were given a pamphlet entitled *Living with the Culture of Control*, which noted that one of the physical

problems associated with vomiting was "calluses over knuckles if hands are used to induce vomiting" (Women's Health Project, 1992, 7).

3. Catherine of Sienna, called the "holy anorexic," was unable to vomit spontaneously and so was compelled "to let a fine straw or some such thing be pushed far down her throat to make her vomit." This became part of her daily routine until the end of her life (Rampling 1985, 91).
4. Medical discussions of the links between anorexia and asceticism can be found in Bruch 1973, 11–13; Crisp 1980, 5, 10; Mogul 1980; and Rampling 1985.
5. Kristeva and Douglas classify semen as nonpolluting (Douglas 1984, 125; Kristeva 1982, 71). Findings of this research highlight the opposite, for women in this project found the viscosity and taste of semen intensely disgusting and polluting. Those I spoke to about oral sex shuddered at the thought of swallowing semen, and it was, as Bettina described, "matter out of place": "It has that mucus quality and it's cloudy and it reminds me of someone with a cold (laughs)—don't even think about it—it's horrible. I have swallowed it before but I prefer not to because then I start thinking about its way—its journey through my system. It kind of to me seems a bit like when someone drinks their own urine—there's something not right about this. . . . I don't like my own bodily fluids."
6. I do not wish to suggest that all men who have anorexia are homosexual (as Crisp and Toms 1972 reports), as this would only compound the taken-for-granted assumption that anorexia is a "feminized" condition. The more interesting question concerning men with eating disorders and their sexual orientation would concern with their own perceptions of identity, connection, and displacement in fields of relatedness that privilege heterosexuality. While little research explores eating disorders among men, some studies suggest that homosexuality is a risk factor for developing eating disorders (Russell and Keel 2002; Weltzin et al. 2005).
7. The American Psychiatric Association (APA) reports: "Sexual abuse has been reported in 20–50% of patients with bulimia nervosa and those with anorexia nervosa, although sexual abuse may be more common in patients with bulimia nervosa than in those with the restricting subtype of anorexia nervosa. Childhood sexual abuse histories are reported more often in women with eating disorders than in women from the general population" (APA 2000, 28).
8. I suspect that if I had specifically asked every participant, this number might have been higher.
9. There are few long-term follow-up clinical studies of recovery (psychiatric and psychological) from anorexia nervosa (see, for example, Herzog 1988; Zipfel et al. 2000). Despite the varying definitions of "recovery," most of these studies agree that "the percentage of individuals with anorexia nervosa who fully recover is modest" (APA 2000, 23).
10. While recounting horrific events or "strange" practices, some participants laughed. Kristeva notes that "laughing is a way of placing or displacing abjection" (1982, 8).
11. Ellen similarly described her experiences of being "fed" via a nasogastric tube as one of "violation": "My stay in the hospital was very scary because it was the first time I was getting any sort of real treatment and I had a tube down my nose and that really, really scared me, to tell you the truth. . . . I felt violated. I was angry with having this food coming in me that I had no control over and I was scared."
12. In a chapter on disgust and shame, Probyn begins: "Like many, I spent much of my childhood feeling disgusting" (2000, 125). She then immediately writes about her experiences of anorexia.

13. Liu similarly opens her autobiography *Solitaire* (1979) with an account of a rape by two boys that took place during a holiday family visit.

14. Any mention of naturopaths during ward rounds at one major hospital brought sighs of exasperation, rolling of eyes, and disparaging comments from attending staff. Naturopaths were seen as assisting in obsessions about certain foods. Psychiatrists' fears are validated on a pro-anorexia Web site, where the benefits of cleansing from a detoxification diet are highlighted.

15. Although Bettina presented herself as demure and morally pure, her conversations were often interspersed with humorous (and whispered) stories about her sexual relationships with men. She characterized herself as having "a problem" with sex; while she has some pleasure from sex, she doesn't like the thought of men "entering" her and has never "let herself go" and had an orgasm. The thought of bodily processes during sex, of vaginal secretions and semen inside of her, disgusts her.

16. Early feminist writing on anorexia argued that it was a form of female social protest against oppressive and contradictory roles of femininity (Chernin 1986; Orbach 1978, 1986). Within this formulation, protesting against the digestive system could have been taken as a humorous extension, as one of Margaret Atwood's characters in *The Edible Woman* wryly points out:

    > Says Marian who can't eat anymore prior to her wedding; "I'm sorry I don't know why I do it, but I can't seem to help it." She was thinking, maybe I can say I'm on a diet.
    >
    > "Oh," said Duncan, "you're probably representative of modern youth, rebelling against the system; though it isn't considered orthodox to begin with the digestive system." (1980, 192)

17. Possible causes for amenorrhea have been related to physiological conditions such as "endocrine dysfunction (hypothalamic dysfunction or to dysfunctions of the hypo-thalamic-pituitary-ovarian axis)" (Malson and Ussher 1996, 506).

18. Martin has extensively documented the separation of self from body that women describe when they talk about menstruation, menopause, and birth (1987, 77–91).

19. "Better out than in" is a common phrase used to joke about emitting bodily gas (burping and farting) and emotions. It is a phrase that pays homage to the body as a contained and bounded unit that needs to rid itself of wastes.

20. Becker notes that the connection between danger and fertility has been well traversed in ethnographic fieldwork (1995, 94). Meigs (1984), for example, has written about female reproductive powers and their association with contamination, potency, and danger in the Highlands of New Guinea. Weiner has also shown this relationship in the Trobriand Islands, where female power is contained in the ability to regenerate human beings (1976, 228–229). The embodied, cosmological potency of this power meant that "women represent sexuality and fertility, but also danger" (193).

CHAPTER 7 BE-COMING CLEAN

1. John Gray's (2006) *Domestic Mandala: Architecture of Lifeworlds in Nepal* is one striking exception to this tendency of ethnographers to ignore homes.

2. Some clinicians argue that obsessive symptoms are the result of food restriction, as evidenced by the infamous Minnesota experiment of 1950 (Keys, Broezek, and Henschel 1950; Sorokin 1941, 31), in which thirty-six male volunteers were observed

as they fasted over several months. The effects of starvation on these men are still used to explain symptoms of anorexia nervosa amongst women, as this extract from a recent treatment manual describes: "Some of the clinical features associated with eating disorders may result from malnutrition or semi-starvation. Studies of volunteers who have submitted to semistarvation and semistarved prisoners of war report the development of food preoccupation, food hoarding, abnormal taste preferences, binge eating, and other disturbances of appetite regulation as well as symptoms of depression, obsessionality, apathy, irritability and other personality changes" (APA 2000, 20). While not disagreeing with the physical effects of starvation, I do take issue with the assumption that men's experiences can be transposed to all bodies. "Male" is taken as the generic, as the standard template from which all other experiences can be explained. The fact that 95 percent of people diagnosed with anorexia are women seems to be overlooked in this research. Gender cannot be omitted from research into eating disorders.

3. This word "ritual" was used frequently by clinicians and participants to denote idiosyncratic structure and routine of behaviors.
4. The cover of the program of Sydney Theatre Company's production of *What Is the Matter with Mary Jane* emphasizes the connections between anorexia and private domestic spaces. It depicts a red toilet/bathroom door with an Engaged sign on it. The title of the play was taken from A. A. Milne's poem "Rice Pudding," and the first verse is written in small, black handwriting on the toilet door: "What is the matter with Mary Jane? / She's crying with all her might and main, / And she won't eat her dinner—rice pudding again— / What is the matter with Mary Jane?"
5. Mandy Thomas (1999, 49) also makes this point in her ethnography of Vietnamese Australians living in transition.
6. Eva Sallis, in her novel about an Arab woman's feelings of displacement in her new Australian home, describes the breakdown of the relationship between the mother and daughter in which food is central to their connection/disconnection.
7. This cultural construction of privacy is an important aspect of anorexia. How would many of the participants in this book practice anorexia in the houses that Carsten describes in Langkawi, which are characterized by a general lack of division of interior space (Carsten and Hugh-Jones 1995, 113)? Houses usually consist of a hearth and one main room, and individual household members do not have their own daytime space.
8. The politics was played out when the film engendered cries of obscenity and disgust, counterbalanced by appreciation of its voluptuous visual aesthetics.
9. Too often the dichotomies of private and public are applied to hospitals with little acknowledgment of the multiple ways in which these concepts operate in such as a space. Within public (for example, government-funded) hospitals there are a myriad of private and public spaces—operating rooms, for example, are the quintessential spaces of privacy that are never seen or accessed by the general public (unless one is undergoing surgery, and even then one's memories of such spaces are anesthetized).
10. Succeeding citations of this source will appear in the text as page numbers in parentheses.
11. Vigarello notes that "the most diverse substances could be used to saturate the skin. Salt, oil and wax, in particular, would all serve to stop up the pores. The body was even coated as if it were a glossy and protected object" (1988, 16).

12. Foucault similarly traces the history of hygiene as a "regime of health for populations [that] entails a certain number of authoritarian medical interventions and controls" (1980, 175). Like Vigarello's, his focus is on the discursive powers of collective hygiene; on families, hospitals, public/urban spaces, and public health. Despite Foucault's emphasis on the role of parents in "good health"—"obligations of a physical kind (care, contact, hygiene, cleanliness, attentive proximity), suckling of children by their mothers, clean clothing, physical exercise to ensure the proper development of the organism" (172)—he does not extend his discussion into the realms of gender or everyday practice.
13. Murcott's 1993 ethnographic study of twenty young women in a South Wales valley talking about the body management of their infants similarly notes the extraordinary emphasis placed on mothers concerning purity and pollution.
14. In her hospital case notes a psychiatrist noted that Grace's orange palms were caused by sensitivity to the beta-carotene in orange vegetables (such as carrots).
15. The introduction to the most recent edition of this book (2000) describes Beeton's work as "one of the major publishing success stories of the nineteenth century, selling over 60, 000 copies in its first year of publication in 1861, and nearly two million by 1868. . . . [As] the most famous English cookery book ever published . . . it stands . . . in the nation's imagination as a bastion of traditional English fare and solid English values" (Humble 2000, vi).
16. In the late 1880s hygienists in the United Kingdom concentrated on teaching hygiene to young women in schools. "From 1882," Forty writes, "all girls in London Boarding Schools had been given some instruction in basic cookery and housework to equip them for domestic service (their most likely occupation upon leaving school) as well as to prepare them for future marriage" (1986, 161).
17. As Forty notes, English school textbooks such as Hood's *Fighting Dirty* (1916) drew on the simplistic metaphors of warfare and racism to promote the dangers of dirt: "Its premise was that the allies of disease, which were dirt, flies, breathing through the mouth, spitting, impure air and darkness, could be identified with the forces of evil. Through the allegory of warfare, hygiene was presented as a constant battle, with the body as a fort always in danger of attack by enemy germs (represented in illustrations by German soldiers). Only by constant vigilance against the forces of disease could the body survive and be victorious" (Forty 1986, 168).
18. In the acknowledgments to *Wasted*, Hornbacher thanks her family "for not throwing a fit about the airing of family laundry in public" (1999, 298).
19. Desjarlais notes that in Helambu, expressing anger, grief, and heartache to family members does not come easily: "Despite the social value of hiding feelings from the gaze of others, *Yolmo wa* consider it important to clean the heart free of pollutants by 'talking' them out at home. The Buddhist aesthetic of purity contributes to this idea: the heart needs to be cleansed of such thoughts, as if they were dirty or harmful, just as ghosts need to be "thrown" and pollution "cut" from the body" (1992, 116).
20. See also Malson, who, in a play on Pink Floyd's lyrics, entitles a short chapter "(Un) comfortably Numb: Purging, Purity and Emptiness" (1998, 166).
21. Ellen West, one of Binswanger's "anorexic cases," similarly wrote in her diaries: "I don't understand myself at all. It is terrible not to understand yourself. *I confront myself as a strange person*. . . . I long to be violated—*and indeed I do violence to myself every hour*" (Binswanger 1958, 254–255, emphasis in original).

22. Malson notes a similar response from one of her participants: "Whilst purging is construed as purifying it may also, paradoxically, be construed as shameful. Nicki, for example, did not like to say that she takes laxatives and avoided using the word. She also avoided any detailed description of their effects—they make you "sick or whatever"—and both her and Cathy's construal of their effects as cleansing might be read as concealing their defecation-inducing properties" (1998, 167).

CHAPTER 8 REIMAGINING ANOREXIA

1. "Lose weight now, ask me how," is the motto of the Herbalife business, an U.S.-based company that sells weight-loss tablets to a worldwide distribution network. The founder, Mark Hughes, dedicated his life to "bringing the finest weight loss, nutritional and personal care products to people around the world." On May 21, 2000, Hughes was found dead at his home following ingestion of a lethal mix of antidepressants and alcohol (*Weekend Australian*, October 7–8, 2000).
2. This community organization publicized a number of Web sites (such as about-face.org and adiosbarbie.com) that exposed negative media images of women.

REFERENCES

Abram, D. 1997. *The Spell of the Sensuous: Perception and Language in a More-Than-Human World.* New York: Vintage Books.

Abu-Lughod, L. 1986. *Veiled Sentiments: Honour and Poetry in a Bedouin Society.* Berkeley: University of California Press.

——. 1991. "Writing against culture." In *Recapturing Anthropology: Working in the Present*, ed. R. Fox, 137–162. Santa Fe, N.M.: School of American Research Press.

——. 1993. *Writing Women's Worlds: Bedouin Stories.* Berkeley: University of California Press.

——. 1995. "A tale of two pregnancies." In *Women Writing Culture*, ed. R. Behar and D. Gordon, 339–350. Berkeley: University of California Press.

Abu-Lughod, L., and C. Lutz. 1990. "Introduction: Emotion, discourse, and the politics of everyday life." In *Language and the Politics of Emotion*, ed. C. Lutz and L. Abu-Lughod, 1–24. Cambridge: Cambridge University Press.

Alexeyeff, K. 2004. "Love food: exchange and sustenance among the Cook Islands diaspora." *Australian Journal of Anthropology* 15: 68–79.

American Psychiatric Association. 1980. *Diagnostic and Statistical Manual of Mental Disorders.* Washington, D.C: American Psychiatric Association.

——. 1987. *Diagnostic and Statistical Manual of Mental Disorders.* 3rd ed., rev. Washington, D.C: American Psychiatric Association.

——. 1994. *Diagnostic and Statistical Manual of Mental Disorders.* 4th ed. Washington, D.C: American Psychiatric Association.

American Psychiatric Association and Work Group on Eating Disorders. 2000. *Practice Guideline for the Treatment of Patients with Eating Disorders.* Washington, D.C.: American Psychiatric Association.

Angel, M., and Z. Sofia. 1996. "Cooking up: intestinal economies and the aesthetics of specular orality." *Cultural Studies* 10(3): 464–483.

Appadurai, A., ed. 1986. *The Social Life of Things: Commodities in Cultural Perspective.* Cambridge: Cambridge University Press.

Ariss, R. 1993. "Performing anger: Emotion in strategic responses to AIDS." *Australian Journal of Anthropology* 4: 18–30.

Aronson, N. 1982a. "Nutrition as a social problem: A case study of entrepreneurial strategy in science." *Social Problems* 29: 474–487.

——. 1982b. "Social definitions of entitlement: Food needs 1885–1920." *Media, Culture and Society* 4: 51–61.

Atwood, M. 1980. *The Edible Woman.* London: Virago. (First published 1969, HarperCollins.)

Austin, S. 1999. "Fat, loathing and public health: The complicity of science in a culture of disordered eating." *Culture, Medicine and Psychiatry* 23(23): 245–268.

Bachelard, G. 1969. *The Poetics of Space.* Boston: Beacon Press.

Bakhtin, M. 1984. *Rabelais and His World.* Trans. H. Iswolsky. Bloomington: Indiana University Press. (First published 1968, MIT Press.)

Banks, C. 1992. "'Culture' in culture-bound syndromes: The case of anorexia nervosa." *Social Science and Medicine* 34(8): 867–884.

Barrett, R. 1988. "Clinical writing and the documentary construction of schizophrenia." *Culture, Medicine and Psychiatry* 12(3): 265–299.

——. 1996. *The Psychiatric Team and the Social Definition of Schizophrenia.* New York: Cambridge University Press.

Barth, F. 1975. *Ritual and Knowledge among the Baktaman of New Guinea.* New Haven: Yale University Press.

Bartky, S. 1988. "Foucault, femininity and the modernization of patriarchal power." In *Feminism and Foucault: Reflections on Resistance*, ed. I. Diamond and L. Quinby, 61–86. Boston: Northeastern University Press.

Battaglia, D. 1997. "Ambiguating agency: The case of Malinowski's ghost." *American Anthropologist* 99(3): 505–510.

Baudelaire, C. 1975. *Selected Poems.* Trans. J. Richardson. Harmondsworth: Penguin.

Baum, A., and E. Goldner. 1995. "Stealing and eating disorders: A review." *Harvard Review of Psychiatry* 3: 210–221.

Becker, A. 1995. *Body, Self and Society: The View from Fiji.* Philadelphia: University of Pennsylvania Press.

——. 2004a. "Television, disordered eating, and young women in Fiji: Negotiating body image and identity during rapid social change." *Culture, Medicine and Psychiatry* 28(4): 533–559.

——. 2004b. "New global perspectives on eating disorders." *Culture, Medicine and Psychiatry* 28(4): 433–437.

Beeton, I. 1907. *Mrs Beeton's Book of Household Management.* London: S. O. Beeton.

Bell, D. 1998. *Ngarrindjeri Wurruwarrin: A World That Is, Was, and Will Be.* North Melbourne: Spinifex Press.

Bell, R. M. 1985. *Holy Anorexia.* Chicago: University of Chicago Press.

Bellman, B. 1984. *The Language of Secrecy: Symbols and Metaphors in Poro Ritual.* New Brunswick: Rutgers University Press.

Bemis-Vitousek, K. 1997. "Developing motivation for change in individuals with eating disorders." In *Challenge the Body Culture Conference Proceedings.* Brisbane: Queensland University of Technology.

Ben-Tovim, D., K. Walker, P. Gilchrist, R. Freeman, R. Kalucy, and A. Esterman. 2001. "Outcome in patients with eating disorders: A 5-year study." *Lancet* 357: 1254–1257.

Bhabha, H. 1990. "The other question: Difference, discrimination, and the discourse of colonialism." In *Out There: Marginalized and Contemporary Cultures*, ed. R. Ferguson, M. Gever, T. T. Minh-ha, and C. West, 71–81. Cambridge: MIT Press.

——. 1996. "Culture's in-between." In *Questions of Cultural Identity*, ed. S. Hall and P. du Gay, 53–60. London: Sage.

Binswanger, L. 1958. "The case of Ellen West: An anthropological-clinical study." In *Existence: A New Dimension in Psychiatry and Psychology*, ed. R. May, E. Angel, and H. Ellenberger, 237–364. New York: Basic Books.

Bok, S. 1982. *Secrets.* Oxford: Oxford University Press.

Bordo, S. 1988. "Anorexia nervosa: Psychopathology as the crystallization of culture." In *Feminism and Foucault*, ed. I. Diamond and L. Quinby, 87–117. Boston: Northeastern University Press.

——. 1989. "The body and the reproduction of femininity: A feminist appropriation of Foucault." In *Gender/Body/Knowledge: Feminist Reconstructions of Being and Knowing*, ed. A. Jagger and S. Bordo, 13–33. New Brunswick: Rutgers University Press.

——. 1990. "Reading the slender body." In *Body/Politics: Women and the Discourses of Science*, ed. M. Jacobus, E. Fox Keller, and S. Shuttleworth, 83–112. London and New York: Routledge.

Bourdieu, P. 1975. "The specificity of the scientific field and the social conditions of the progress of reason." *Social Science Information* 14(6): 19–47.

——. 1977. *Outline of a Theory of Practice*. Trans. R. Nice. Cambridge: Cambridge University Press.

——. 1984. *Distinction: A Social Critique of the Judgement of Taste*. Trans. R. Nice. London: Routledge and Kegan Paul.

——. 1985. "The social space and the genesis of groups." *Theory and Society* 14: 723–744.

——. 1990. *In Other Words: Essays towards a Reflexive Sociology*. Trans. M. Adamson. Stanford, Calif.: Stanford University Press.

——. 1991. *Language and Symbolic Power*. Trans. G. Raymond and M. Adamson. Cambridge: Polity Press.

Bourdieu, P., and A. Accardo, eds. 1999. *The Weight of the World: Social Suffering in Contemporary Society*. Stanford, Calif.: Stanford University Press.

Bourdieu, P., and L. Wacquant. 1992. *An Invitation to Reflexive Sociology*. Chicago and London: University of Chicago Press.

Bray, A. 1994. "The edible woman: Reading/eating disorders and femininity." *Media Information Australia* 72: 4–10.

——. 1996. "The anorexic body: Reading disorders." *Cultural Studies* 10(3): 413–430.

Bray, A., and C. Colebrook. 1998. "The haunted flesh: Corporeal feminism and the politics of (dis)embodiment." *Signs: Journal of Women in Culture and Society* 24(1): 35–67.

Brown, K. M. 1991. *Mama Lola: A Vodou Priestess in Brooklyn*. Berkeley: University of California Press.

Bruch, H. 1973. *Eating Disorders: Obesity, Anorexia Nervosa and the Person Within*. New York: Basic Book.

——. 1978. *The Golden Cage: The Enigma of Anorexia Nervosa*. Cambridge: Harvard University Press.

Brumberg, J. 1988. *Fasting Girls: The Emergence of Anorexia Nervosa as a Modern Disease*. Cambridge, Mass.: Harvard University Press.

Buckley, T., and A. Gottleib. 1988. "Introduction: A critical appraisal of theories of menstrual symbolism." In *Blood Magic: The Anthropology of Menstruation*, ed. T. Buckley and A. Gottleib, 3–53. Berkeley: University of California Press.

Burke, T. 1996. *Lifebuoy Men, Lux Women: Commodification, Consumption and Cleanliness in Modern Zimbabwe*. Durham, N.C., and London: Duke University Press.

Butler, J. 1990. *Gender Trouble: Feminism and the Subversion of Identity*. New York and London: Routledge.

——. 1993. *Bodies That Matter: On the Discursive Limits of 'Sex.'* London: Routledge.

Butler, R. and H. Parr. 1999. *Mind and Body Spaces: Geographies of Illness, Impairment and Disability*. London and New York: Routledge.

Bynum, C. 1987. *Holy Feast and Holy Fast: The Religious Significance of Food to Medieval Women*. Berkeley: University of California Press.

Cameron, P., K. Willi, and D. Richter. 1997. "Working with people with eating disorders: How do professional attitudes affect approaches to early intervention?" *Australian Journal of Primary Health—Interchange* 3(2, 3): 23–31.

Caplan, P. 1994. *Feasts, fasts, famine: Food for thought*. Berg Occasional Papers in Anthropology. Oxford: Berg.

Caputo, V. 2000. "At 'home' and 'away': Reconfiguring the field for late twentieth-century anthropology." In *Constructing the Field: Ethnographic Fieldwork in the Contemporary World*, ed. V. Amit, 19–31. London: Routledge.

Carrithers, M., S. Collins, and S. Lukes, eds. 1985. *The Category of the Person: Anthropology, Philosophy, History*. Cambridge: Cambridge University Press.

Carsten, J. 1995. "The substance of kinship and the heat of the hearth: Feeding, personhood, and relatedness among Malays in Pulau Langkawi." *American Ethnologist* 22(2): 223–241.

——. 1997. *The Heat of the Hearth: The Process of Kinship in a Malay Fishing Community*. Oxford: Oxford University Press.

——. 2000a. "Introduction: Cultures of relatedness." In *Cultures of Relatedness: New Approaches to the Study of Kinship*, ed. J. Carsten, 1–36. Cambridge: Cambridge University Press.

——, ed. 2000b. *Cultures of Relatedness: New Approaches to the Study of Kinship*. Cambridge: Cambridge University Press.

——. 2004. *After Kinship*. Cambridge: Cambridge University Press.

Carsten, J., and S. Hugh-Jones, eds. 1995. *About the House: Levi-Strauss and Beyond*. Cambridge: Cambridge University Press.

Carter, P. 1987. *The Road to Botany Bay: An Essay in Spatial History*. Boston: Faber and Faber.

Celermajer, D. 1987. "Submission and rebellion: Anorexia and a feminism of the body." *Australian Feminist Studies* 5: 57–70.

Chakrabarty, D. 1994. "Embodying freedom: Gandhi and the body of the public man in India." *Australian Cultural History* 13: 100–110.

Chernin, K. 1986. *The Hungry Self: Daughters and Mothers, Eating and Identity*. London: Virago Press.

Citoys, F. 1623. *Avis sur la nature de la peste*. Paris.

Claude-Pierre, P. 1997. *The Secret Language of Eating Disorders*. New York: Random House.

Clifford, J. 1990. "On collecting art and culture." In *Out There: Marginalization and Contemporary Cultures*, ed. R. Ferguson, M. Gever, T. Minh-ha, and C. West, 141–169. New York: MIT Press.

——. 1992. "Traveling cultures." In *Cultural Studies*, ed. L. Grossberg, C. Nelson, and P. Treichler, 96–116. New York: Routledge.

——. 1997. *Routes: Travel and Translation in the Late Twentieth Century*. Cambridge: Harvard University Press.

Clifford, J., and G. Marcus. 1986. *Writing Culture: The Poetics and Politics of Ethnography*. Berkeley: University of California Press.

Cohen, A., ed. 2000a. *Signifying Identities: Anthropological Perspectives on Boundaries and Contested Values*. London: Routledge.

——. 2000b. "Introduction: Discriminating relations: Identity, boundary and authenticity." In *Signifying Identities: Anthropological Perspectives on Boundaries and Contested Values*, ed. A. Cohen, 1–13. London: Routledge.

Coleman, S., and P. Collins, eds. 2005. *Locating the Field: Space, Place and Context in Anthropology*. New York: Berg.

Coopman, V. 1995. "The history/vision of 'food without fear.'" Paper presented to the Brisbane Eating Disorders and Body Image Conference, Brisbane.

Corbin, A. 1996. *The Foul and the Fragrant: Odor and the Social Imagination*. London: Papermac.

Cosman, B. 1986. "Bloodletting as purging behavior." *American Journal of Psychiatry* 143(9): 1188–1189.

Counihan, C. 1999. *The Anthropology of Food and Body: Gender, Meaning and Power*. New York and London: Routledge.

Coveney, J. 1998. "The government and ethics of health promotion: The importance of Michel Foucault." *Health Education Research* 13(3): 459–468.

——. 1999. "The science and spirituality of nutrition." *Critical Public Health* 9(1): 23–37.

——. 2000. *Food, Morals, and Meaning: The Pleasure and Anxiety of Eating*. London and New York: Routledge.

——. 2008. "The government of girth." *Health Sociology Review* 17(2): 199–213.

Cowan, R. 1976. "Two washes in the morning and a bridge party at night: The American housewife between the wars." *Women's Studies* 3(2): 147–172.

Crisp, A. 1980. *Anorexia Nervosa: Let Me Be*. London: Academic Press.

Crisp, A., and D. Toms. 1972. "Primary anorexia or weight phobia in the male: Report on 13 cases." *British Medical Journal* 1: 334–338.

Crook, T. 2007. *Anthropological Knowledge, Secrecy and Bolivip, Papua New Guinea: Exchanging Skin*. Oxford: Oxford University Press.

Crossley, M. 2002. "The perils of health promotion and the 'barebacking' backlash." *Health* 6(1): 47–68.

Crow, S., P. Keel, and D. Kendall. 1998. "Eating disorders and insulin-dependent diabetes mellitus." *Psychosomatics* 39(3): 233–243.

Csordas, T. 1990. "Embodiment as a paradigm for anthropology." *Ethos* 18(1): 5–47.

——, ed. 1994. *Embodiment and Experience: The Existential Ground of Culture and Self*. Cambridge: Cambridge University Press.

Daluiski, A., B. Rahbar, and R. Meals. 1997. "Russell's sign: Subtle hand changes in patients with bulimia nervosa." *Clinical Orthopaedics*, October, 107–109.

Daniel, E. 1984. *Fluid Signs: Being a Person the Tamil Way*. Berkeley: University of California Press.

Davis, C., S. Kaptein, A. Kaplan, M. Olmstead, and D. Woodside. 1998. "Obsessionality in anorexia nervosa: The moderating effects of exercise." *Psychosomatic Medicine* 60(2): 192–197.

de Certeau, M. 1984. *The Practice of Everyday Life*. Berkeley: University of California Press.

Deleuze, G. 1987. *Dialogues*. Trans. H. Tomlinson and G. Burchill. London: Verso.

Dennis, S. 2007. *Police Beat: The Emotional Power of Music in Police Work*. New York: Cambria Press.

Derrida, J. 1976. *Of Grammatology*. Trans. Gayatri Spivak. Baltimore: Johns Hopkins University Press.

——. 1981. *Positions*. Chicago: University of Chicago Press.

Desjarlais, R. 1992. *Body and Emotion: The Aesthetics of Illness and Healing in the Nepal Himalayas*. Philadelphia: University of Pennsylvania Press.

——. 1996a. "Struggling along." In *Things As They Are: New Directions in Phenomenological Anthropology*, ed. M. Jackson, 70–93. Bloomington and Indianapolis: Indiana University Press.

——. 1996b. "The office of reason: On the politics of language and agency in a shelter for 'the homeless mentally ill.'" *American Ethnologist* 23(4): 880–900.

——. 2003. *Sensory Biographies: Lives and Deaths among Nepal's Yolmo Buddhists*. London: University of California Press.

Devisch, R. 1990. "The human body as a vehicle for emotions among the Yaka of Zaire." In *Personhood and Agency: The Experience of Self and Other in African Cultures*, ed. M. Jackson and I. Karp, 115–133. Washington, D.C.: Smithsonian Institution Press.

Diamond, I., and L. Quinby, eds. 1988. *Feminism and Foucault: Reflections on Resistance.* Boston: Northeastern University Press.

Dias, K. 2003. "The Ana sanctuary: Women's pro-anorexia narratives in cyberspace." *Journal of International Women's Studies* 4(2): 31–45.

Dollimore, J. 1998. *Death, Desire, and Loss in Western Culture.* New York: Routledge.

Donzelot, J. 1979. *The Policing of Families.* New York: Pantheon Press.

Douglas, M. 1984. *Purity and Danger.* Rpt. of 1966 ed. London: Ark.

———. 1973. *Natural Symbols: Explorations in Cosmology.* Harmondsworth: Penguin.

———. 1975. *Implicit Meanings: Essays in Anthropology.* London: Routledge and Kegan Paul.

———. 1987. *How Institutions Think.* Syracuse, N.Y.: Syracuse University Press.

Dovey, K. 1985. "Homes and homelessness." In *Home Environments*, ed. I. Altman and C. Werner, 33–61. New York: Plenum Press.

Eckermann, L. 1994. "Self-starvation and binge-purging: Embodied selfhood/sainthood." *Australian Cultural History* 13: 82–99.

———. 1997. "Foucault, embodiment and gendered subjectivities: The case of voluntary self-starvation." In *Foucault, Health and Medicine*, ed. A. Petersen and R. Bunton, 151–169.

Edwards, J. 1993. "Explicit connections: Ethnographic inquiry in north-west England." In *Technologies of Procreation: Kinship in the Age of Assisted Conception*, ed. J. Edwards, S. Franklin, E. Hirsch, F. Price, and M. Strathern, 42–66. Manchester: Manchester University Press.

———. 2000. *Born and Bred: Idioms of Kinship and New Reproductive Technologies in England.* Oxford: Oxford University Press.

Edwards, J., and M. Strathern. 2000. "Including our own." In *Cultures of Relatedness: New Approaches to the Study of Kinship*, ed. J. Carsten, 149–166. Cambridge: Cambridge University Press.

Ehrenreich, B. 1990. *Fear of Falling: The Inner Life of the Middle Class.* New York: Harper Collins.

Elias, N. 1982. *The History of Manners.* Vol. 1, *The Civilizing Process.* Trans. E. Jephcott. New York: Pantheon.

Ellman, M. 1990. "Eliot's abjection." In *Abjection, Melancholia, and Love*, ed. J. Fletcher and A. Benjamin, 178–200. London: Routledge.

Epstein, D. 1993. "On affect and musical motion." In *Psychoanalytic Explorations in Music*, 2nd. series, ed. S. Feder, R. Karmel, and G. Pollock, 91–124. Madison, Conn.: International Universities Press.

Ernst, T. 1990. "Mates, wives and children: An exploration of concepts of relatedness in Australian culture." *Social Analysis* 27: 110–129.

Evans-Pritchard, E. 1976. *Witchcraft, Oracles and Magic among the Azande.* Oxford: Clarendon Press.

Fabian, J. 1983. *Time and the Other: How Anthropology Makes Its Object.* New York: Columbia University Press.

Fairburn, C., and P. Harrison. 2003. "Eating disorders." *Lancet* 361: 407–416.

Favazza, A. 1996. *Bodies under Siege: Self-Mutilation and Body Modification in Culture and Psychiatry.* Baltimore: Johns Hopkins University Press.

Feld, S., and K. Basso, eds. 1996. *Senses of Place.* Santa Fe, N.M.: School of American Research Press.

Finn, S., M. Hartmann, G. Leon, and L. Lawson. 1986. "Eating disorders and sexual abuse: Lack of confirmation for a clinical hypothesis." *International Journal of Eating Disorders* 5: 1051–1060.

Foley, D. E. 1990. *Learning Capitalist Culture: Deep in the Heart of Tejas*. Philadelphia: University of Pennsylvania Press.

Forty, A. 1986. *Objects of Desire*. London: Thames and Hudson.

Foucault, M. 1972. *The Archeology of Knowledge and the Discourse on Language*. New York: Pantheon Books.

———. 1973. *The Birth of the Clinic*. Trans. A. Sheridan. London: Tavistock Publications.

———. 1977. *Discipline and Punish: The Birth of the Prison*. Trans. A. Sheridan. London: Allen Lane.

———. 1980. *Power/Knowledge*. London: Harvester.

———. 1990. *The History of Sexuality*. Vol. 2, *The Use of Pleasure*. Trans. R. Hurley. New York: Vintage Books.

Fox, N., K. Ward, and A. O'Rourke. 2005. "Pro-anorexia, weight-loss drugs and the Internet: An 'anti-recovery' explanatory model of anorexia." *Sociology of Health and Illness* 27(7): 944–971.

Frank, A. 1990. "Bringing bodies back in: A decade in review." *Theory, Culture and Society* 7: 131–162.

Frankenberg, R. 1988. "Gramsci, culture, and medical anthropology: Kundry and Parsifal? or rat's tail to sea serpent." *Medical Anthropology Quarterly* 2(4): 324–337.

Franklin, S. 1997. *Embodied Progress: A Cultural Account of Assisted Conception*. London: Routledge.

———. 2003. "Re-thinking nature-culture: Anthropology and the new genetics." *Anthropological Theory* 3(1): 65–85.

Frazer, J. 1959. *The New Golden Bough: A New Abridgment of the Classic Work by Sir James George Frazer. Ed. T Gaster*. New York: Phillips.

Freud, A. 1958. "Adolescence." *Psychoanalytic Study of the Child* 13: 255–278.

Friedman, S. 1998. *Mappings: Feminism and the Cultural Geographies of Encounter*. Princeton: Princeton University Press.

Fuery, P. 1995. *Theories of Desire*. Melbourne: Melbourne University Press.

Garrett, C. 1992. "Anorexia as personal and social ritual." Working Papers in Women's Studies, 6. Women's Research Center: University of Western Sydney, Nepean, Sydney.

———. 1998. *Beyond Anorexia*. Cambridge: Cambridge University Press.

Gauthier, D., and C. Forsyth. 1999. "Bareback Sex, Bug Chasers, and the Gift of Death." *Deviant Behavior* 20(1): 85–100.

Geertz, C. 1973. *The Interpretation of Cultures: Selected Essays*. New York: Basic Books.

Gell, A. 1977. "Magic, perfume, dream . . ." In *Symbols and Sentiments: Cross-cultural Studies in Symbolism*, ed. I. M. Lewis, 25–38. London: Academic Press.

Geurts, K. 2002. *Culture and the Senses: Bodily Ways of Knowing in an African Community*. Berkeley: University of California Press.

Giddens, A. 1991. *Modernity and Self-Identity: Self and Society in the Late Modern Age*. Cambridge: Polity.

Giles, D. 2006. "Constructing identities in cyberspace: The case of eating disorders." *British Journal of Social Psychology* 45: 463–477.

Gilroy, P. 1994. *The Black Atlantic: Modernity and Double Consciousness*. London: Verso.

Glick, L. 1967. "Medicine as an ethnographic category: The Gimi of the New Guinea highlands." *Ethnology* 6: 31–56.

Goldner, E., J. Geller, L. Birmingham, and R. Remick. 2000. "Comparison of shoplifting behaviors in patients with eating disorders, psychiatric control subjects, and undergraduate control subjects." *Canadian Journal of Psychiatry* 45: 471–475.

Good, B. 1994. *Medicine, Rationality, and Experience: An Anthropological Perspective*. Cambridge: Cambridge University Press.

Gooldin, S. 2003. "Fasting women, living skeletons and hunger artists: Spectacles of body and miracles at the turn of a century." *Body and Society* 9(2): 27–53.

———. 2008. "Being anorexic: Hunger, subjectivity and embodied morality." *Medical Anthropology Quarterly* 22(3): 274–296.

Gordon, R. 2000. *Eating Disorders: Anatomy of a Social Epidemic. 2nd. ed.* Boston: Blackwell.

Graham, D. 1997. "Time and the experience of HIV/AIDS: An anthropological study of illness." Honors thesis, Department of Psychiatry, Adelaide University.

Gray, J. 1996. *Domestic Mandala: Architecture of Lifeworlds in Nepal*. Aldershot: Ashgate.

———. 1999. "Open spaces and dwelling places: Being at home on hill farms in the Scottish borders." *American Ethnologist* 26(2): 440–460.

Gremillion, H. 1992. "Psychiatry as social ordering: Anorexia nervosa, a paradigm." *Social Science and Medicine* 35(1): 57–71.

———. 1996. *In Fitness and in Health: Crafting Bodies, Selves, and Families in the Treatment of Anorexia Nervosa*. PhD diss., Department of Cultural Anthropology, Stanford University.

———. 2002. "In fitness and in health: Crafting bodies in the treatment of anorexia nervosa." *Signs: Journal of Women in Culture and Society* 27(2): 381–414.

———. 2003. *Feeding Anorexia: Gender and Power at a Treatment Center*. Durham, N.C.: Duke University Press.

Grieves, L. 1997. "From beginning to start: The Vancouver Anti-Anorexia Anti-Bulimia League." *Gecko: A Journal of Deconstruction and Narrative Ideas on Therapeutic Practice* 2: 78–88.

Grimm, V. 1996. *From Feasting to Fasting, the Evolution of a Sin: Attitudes to Food in Late Antiquity*. London, New York: Routledge.

Grosz, E. 1989. *Sexual Subversions: Three French Feminists*. Sydney: Allen and Unwin.

———. 1990. "The body of signification." In *Abjection, Melancholia, and Love*, ed. J. Fletcher and A. Benjamin, 80–103. New York: Routledge.

———. 1994. *Volatile Bodies: Towards a Corporeal Feminism*. Sydney: Allen and Unwin.

Gupta, A., and J. Ferguson. 1992. "Beyond 'culture': Space, identity and the politics of difference." *Cultural Anthropology* 7(1): 6–23.

———. ed. 1997. *Anthropological Locations: Boundaries and Grounds of Field Science*. London: University of California Press.

Hall, S. 1996. "Introduction: Who needs 'identity'?" In *Questions of Cultural Identity*, ed. S. Hall and P. du Gay, 1–17. New York: Sage.

Hall, S., and P. du Gay, eds. 1996. *Questions of Cultural Identity*. New York: Sage.

Hannerz, U. 2003. "Being there . . . , and there . . . , and there!: Reflections of multi-sited ethnography." *Ethnography* 4(2): 201–216.

———. 2004. *Foreign News: Exploring the World of Foreign Correspondents*. Chicago: University of Chicago Press.

Haraway, D. 1988. "Situated knowledges: The science of question in feminism and the privilege of partial perspective." *Feminist Studies* 14(4): 575–599.

Harker, R., C. Mahar, and C. Wilkes, eds. 1990. *An Introduction to the Work of Pierre Bourdieu*. London: Macmillan Press.

Harris, G. 1989. "Concepts of individual, self and person in description and analysis." *American Anthropologist* 91: 599–612.

Harrison, K. 1997. *The Kiss*. New York: Random House.

Hastrup, K. 1995. *A Passage to Anthropology*. New York: Routledge.

Heidegger, M. 1977. *Basic Writings from Being and Time (1927) to The Task of Thinking (1964).* New York: Harper and Row.

——. 1982. *The Basic Problems of Phenomenology.* Trans. A. Hofstadter. Bloomington: Indiana University Press.

Hepworth, J. 1999. *The Social Construction of Anorexia Nervosa.* London: Sage.

Herdt, G. 1990. "Secret societies and secret collectives." *Oceania* 60(4): 360–381.

Herzfeld, M. 2001. *Anthropology: Theoretical Practice in Culture and Society.* Oxford: Blackwell.

Herzog, W. 1988. "Outcome in anorexia nervosa and bulimia nervosa: A review of the literature." *Journal of Nervous and Mental Disease* 176(3): 131–143.

Herzog, W., H. Deter, W. Fiehn, and E. Petzold. 1997. "Medical findings and predictors of long-term physical outcome in anorexia nervosa: A prospective, 12-year follow-up study." *Psychological Medicine* 27: 269–279.

Hinton, D., D. Howes, and L. Kirmayer. 2008. "The medical anthropology of sensations." *Transcultural Psychiatry* 45(2): 139–141.

Hirsch, E., and M. O'Hanlon, eds. 1995. *The Anthropology of Landscape: Perspectives on Place and Space.* Oxford: Clarendon Press.

Holden, N. 1991. "Adoption and eating disorders: A high-risk group?" *British Journal of Psychiatry* 158: 829–833.

Holy, L. 1996. *Anthropological Perspectives on Kinship.* London: Pluto.

Honkasalo, M. L. 1991. "Medical symptoms: A challenge for semiotic research." *Semiotica* 87(3/4): 251–268.

Hornbacher, M. 1999. *Wasted: A Memoir of Anorexia and Bulimia.* London: Flamingo.

Houppert, K. 1999. *The Curse: Confronting the Last Unmentionable Taboo—Menstruation.* Sydney: Allen and Unwin.

Howes, D., ed. 1991. *The Varieties of Sensory Experience: A Sourcebook in the Anthropology of the Senses.* Toronto: University of Toronto Press.

——. 2003. *Sensual Relations: Engaging the Senses in Culture and Social Theory.* Ann Arbor: University of Michigan Press.

Hoy, S. 1995. *Chasing Dirt: The American Pursuit of Cleanliness.* New York: Oxford University Press.

Humble, N., ed. 2000. *Mrs Beeton's Book of Household Management.* New York: Oxford University Press.

Ingold, T. 1991. "Becoming persons: Consciousness and sociality in human evolution." *Cultural-Dynamics* 4(3): 355–378.

——. ed. 1992. *Language Is the Essence of Culture.* Group for Debates in Anthropological Theory. Department of Social Anthropology, University of Manchester. London: Publishing Solutions.

Iossifides, M. 1992. "Wine: Life's blood and spiritual essence in a Greek Orthodox convent." In *Alcohol, Gender and Culture,* ed. D. Gefou-Madianou, 80–100. New York: Routledge.

Irigaray, L. 1999. *The Forgetting of Air in Martin Heidegger.* Trans. M. B. Mader. London: Athlone Press.

Jackson, M. 1989. *Paths towards a Clearing: Radical Empiricism and Ethnographic Enquiry.* Bloomington: Indiana University Press.

——. 1996. "Introduction: Phenomenology, radical empiricism, and anthropological critique." In *Things As They Are: New Directions in Phenomenological Anthropology,* ed. M. Jackson, 1–50. Bloomington and Indianapolis: Indiana University Press.

——. 1998. *Minima Ethnographica.* Chicago: University of Chicago Press.

Jarry, J., and F. Vaccarino. 1996. "Eating disorder and obsessive compulsive disorder: Neurochemical and phenomenological commonalities." *Journal of Psychiatry and Neuroscience* 21(1): 36–48.

Jenkins, J., and R. Barrett, eds. 2004. *Schizophrenia, Culture and Subjectivity: The Edge of Experience.* Cambridge: Cambridge University Press.

Jenkins, R. 1992. *Pierre Bourdieu.* London: Routledge.

Kafka, F. 1992. "A Hunger Artist." In *The Complete Short Stories of Franz Kafka*, ed. N. Glatzer, 268–277. London: Minerva.

Kapferer, B. 1997. *The Feast of the Sorcerer: Practices of Consciousness and Power.* Chicago: University of Chicago Press.

Katzman, M. 1993. "The pregnant therapist and the eating-disordered woman: The challenge of fertility." *Eating Disorders* 1(1): 17–30.

Katzman, M., and S. Lee. 1997. "Beyond body image: The integration of feminist and transcultural theories in the understanding of self starvation." *International Journal of Eating Disorders* 22: 385–394.

Keys, A., J. Broezek, and A. Henschel. 1950. *The Biology of Human Starvation.* Minneapolis: University of Minnesota Press.

Khare, R. 1980. "Food as nutrition and culture: Notes towards an anthropological methodology." *Social Science Information* 19(3): 519–542.

Kiev, A. 1972. *Transcultural Psychiatry.* New York: Free Press.

Kirmayer, L. 1992. "The body's insistence on meaning: Metaphor as presentation and representation in illness experience." *Medical Anthropology Quarterly* 6(4): 323–346.

Kleinman, A. 1988. *The Illness Narratives: Suffering, Healing and the Human Condition.* New York: Basic Books.

Kok, I. P., and C. S. Tian. 1994. "Susceptibility of Singapore Chinese schoolgirls to anorexia nervosa: Part I (psychological factors)." *Singapore Medical Journal* 35: 481–485.

Kondo, D. 1986. "Dissolution and reconstitution of self: Implications for anthropological epistemology." *Cultural Anthropology* 1:74–88.

Kristeva, J. 1982. *Powers of Horror: An Essay on Abjection.* New York: Columbia University Press.

———. 1984. *Revolution in Poetic Language.* Trans. M. Waller. New York: Columbia University Press.

———. 1990. "An interview with Julia Kristeva: Cultural strangeness and the subject in crisis, with Suzanne Clark and Kathleen Hulley." *Discourse* 13(1): 149–180.

Lacey, J. 1990. "Incest, incestuous fantasy and indecency: A clinical catchment area study of normal weight bulimic women." *British Journal of Psychiatry* 157: 399–403.

Laclau, E. 1990. *New Reflections on the Revolution of Our Time.* London: Verso.

Laderman, C. 1994. "The embodiment of symbols and the acculturation of the anthropologist." In *Embodiment and Experience: The Existential Ground of Culture and Self*, ed. T. Csordas, 183–200. Cambridge: Cambridge University Press.

Laermans, R., and C. Meulders. 1999. "The domestication of laundering." In *At Home: An Anthropology of Domestic Space*, ed. I. Cieraad, 118–129. Syracuse: Syracuse University Press.

Leavitt, J. 1996. "Meaning and feeling in the anthropology of emotions." *American Ethnologist* 23(3): 514–539.

Lechte, J. 1990. *Julia Kristeva.* London: Routledge.

Leder, D. 1990. *The Absent Body.* Chicago: University of Chicago.

Lee, S. 2001. "Fat phobia in anorexia nervosa: Whose obsession is it?" In *Eating Disorders and Cultures in Transition*, ed. M. Nasser, M. Katzman, and R. Gordon, 40–65. London: Routledge.

——. 2004 "Engaging culture: An overdue task for eating disorders research." Culture, Medicine and Psychiatry 28:617–621.

Lee, S., T. Ho, and L. Hsu. 1993. "Fat phobic and non-fat phobic anorexia nervosa—A comparative study of 70 Chinese patients in Hong Kong." *Psychological Medicine* 23: 999–1017.

Leonard, V. 1994. "A Heideggerian Phenomenological Perspective on the Person." In *Interpretive Phenomenology: Embodiment, Caring and Ethics in Health and Illness*, ed. P. Benner, 43–64. Thousand Oaks, Calif.: Sage Publications.

Lester, R. 1995. "Embodied voices: Women's food asceticism and the negotiation of identity." *Ethos* 23(2): 187–222.

——. 1997. "The (dis)embodied self in anorexia nervosa." *Social Science and Medicine* 44(4): 479–489.

——. 2000. "Like a Natural Woman: Celibacy and the Embodied Self in Anorexia Nervosa." In *Celibacy, Culture, and Society: The Anthropology of Sexual Abstinence*, ed. E. J. Sobo and S. Bell, 197–213. Madison: University of Wisconsin Press.

——. 2007. "Critical therapeutics: Cultural politics and clinical reality in two eating disorder treatment centers." *Medical Anthropology Quarterly* 21(4): 369–387.

Lévi-Strauss, C. 1973. *Tristes Tropiques*. Trans. J. Weightman and D. Weightman. London: Jonathon Cape.

——. 1981. *The Naked Man*. Trans. J. Weightman and D. Weightman. Chicago: University of Chicago Press.

Liu, A. 1979. *Solitaire*. New York: Harper and Row.

Lovell, T. 2000. "Thinking feminism with and against Bourdieu." *Feminist Theory* 1(1): 11–32.

Low, S., and D. Lawrence-Zuniga. 2003. *The Anthropology of Space and Place*. Oxford: Blackwell.

Lucas, R. 1999. *Uncommon Lives: An Ethnography of Schizophrenia as Extraordinary Experience*. PhD thesis, Departments of Anthropology and Psychiatry, Adelaide University.

Lucas, R., and R. Barrett. 1995. "Interpreting culture and psychopathology: Primitivist themes in cross-cultural debate." *Culture, Medicine and Psychiatry* 19: 287–326.

Luhrmann, T. 1989a. "The magic of secrecy." *Ethos* 17: 131–165.

——. 1989b. *Persuasions of the Witch's Craft*. Oxford: Blackwell.

Lupton, D. 1994. *Medicine as Culture: Illness, Disease and the Body in Western Societies*. London: Sage.

——. 1996. *Food, the Body, and the Self*. London: Sage.

——. 1997. "Foucault and the medicalization critique." In *Foucault, Health, and Medicine*, ed. A. Petersen and R. Bunton, 94–112. London: Routledge.

Lupton, D., and J. A. Miller. 1992. "Hygiene, cuisine and the product world of early twentieth-century America." In *Incorporations*, ed. J. Crary and S. Kwinter, 497–515. New York: Urzone.

Lutz, C., and L. Abu-Lughod, eds. 1990. *Language and the Politics of Emotion*. Cambridge: Cambridge University Press.

Lutz, C., and G. White. 1986. "The Anthropology of Emotions." *Annual Review of Anthropology* 15: 405–436.

Lynch, M. 1987. "The body: Thin is beautiful." *Arena* 79: 128–145.

Lynch, O. 1990. "The social construction of emotion in India." In *Divine Passions: The Social Construction of Emotion in India*, ed. O. Lynch, 3–37. Berkeley: University of California Press.

Lyotard, J. F. 1984. *The Postmodern Condition: A Report on Knowledge.* Trans. M. Lopez-Morillas and L. Solotaraff. Cambridge, Mass.: Harvard University Press.

MacLeod, S. 1981. *The Art of Starvation.* London: Virago.

MacSween, M. 1993. *Anorexic Bodies: A Feminist and Sociological Perspective on Anorexia Nervosa.* New York: Routledge.

Malinowski, B. 1929. *The Sexual Life of Savages in North-western Melanesia.* New York: Harcourt, Brace and World.

Malson, H. 1997. "Anorexic bodies and the discursive production of feminine excess." In *Body Talk: The Material and Discursive Regulation of Sexuality, Madness and Reproduction*, ed. J. Ussher, 223–245. New York: Routledge.

——. 1998. *The Thin Woman: Feminism, Post-structuralism and the Social Psychology of Anorexia Nervosa.* London: Routledge.

Malson, H., and J. Ussher. 1996. "Bloody women: A discourse analysis of amenorrhea as a symptom of anorexia nervosa." *Feminism and Psychology* 6(4): 505–521.

——. 1997. "Beyond this mortal coil: Femininity, death and discursive constructions of the anorexic body." *Mortality* 2(1): 43–61.

Marcus, G. 1998. *Ethnography through Thick and Thin.* Princeton: Princeton University Press.

——. 1999. "Critical anthropology now: An introduction." In *Critical Anthropology Now*, ed. G. Marcus, 3–28. Santa Fe, N.M.: School of American Research Press.

Marcus, G., and M. Fischer. 1986. *Anthropology as Cultural Critique: An Experimental Moment in the Human Sciences.* Chicago: University of Chicago Press.

Martin, E. 1987. *The Woman in the Body: A Cultural Analysis of Reproduction.* Milton Keynes: Open University Press.

Mauss, M. 1972. *A General Theory of Magic.* Trans. R. Brain. New York: Routledge and Kegan Paul. (First published 1902, Norton.)

McNay, L. 1994. *Foucault: A Critical Introduction.* Cambridge: Polity Press.

——. 1999. "Gender, habitus and the field: Pierre Bourdieu and the limits of reflexivity." *Theory, Culture and Society* 16(1): 95–117.

Meigs, A. 1984. *Food, Sex and Pollution: A New Guinea Religion.* New Brunswick: Rutgers University Press.

——. 1997. "Food as cultural construction." In *Food and Culture*, ed. C. Counihan and P. van Esterik, 95–106. New York: Routledge.

Melville, X. 1983. *The ABC of Eating Disorders: Coping with Anorexia, Bulimia and Compulsive Eating.* London: Sheldon Press.

Mennell, S. 1985. *All Manners of Food: Eating and Taste in England and France from the Middle Ages to the Present.* Oxford: Blackwell.

——. 1991. "On the civilizing of appetite." In *The Body: Social Processes and Cultural Theory*, ed. M. Featherstone, M. Hepworth, and B. Turner, 126–156. London: Sage.

Merleau-Ponty, M. 1973. "Phenomenology and the sciences of man." In *Phenomenology and the Social Sciences*, ed. M. Natanson, 47–108. Evanston: Northwestern University Press.

Messerschmidt, D., ed. 1981. *Anthropologists at Home in North America: Methods and Issues in the Study of One's Own Society.* Cambridge: Cambridge University Press.

Miller, J. 1993. *The Passion of Michel Foucault.* New York: Simon and Schuster.

Miller, W. 1997. *The Anatomy of Disgust.* Cambridge: Harvard University Press.

Mogul, S. 1980. "Asceticism in adolescence and anorexia nervosa." *Psychoanalytic Study of the Child* 35: 155–178.

Moi, T. 1991. "Appropriating Bourdieu: Feminist theory and Pierre Bourdieu's sociology of culture." *New Literary History* 22: 1017–1049.

Moore, H. 1994. *A Passion for Difference*. Bloomington: Indiana University Press.

Moreno, E. 1995. "Rape in the field: Reflections from a survivor." In *Taboo: Sex, Identity and Erotic Subjectivity in Anthropological Fieldwork*, ed. D. Kulick and M. Wilson, 219–250. London: Routledge.

Moulding, N. 2006. "Disciplining the feminine: The reproduction of gender contradictions in the mental health care of women with eating disorders." *Social Science and Medicine* 62(4): 793–804.

Mukai, T. 1989. "A call for our language: Anorexia from within." *Women's Studies International Forum* 12(6): 613–638.

Murcott, A. 1993. "Purity and pollution: Body management and the social place of infancy." In *Body Matters: Essays on the Sociology of the Body*, ed. S. Scott and D. Morgan, 122–134. London: Falmer Press.

Murphy, M. 1997. "Humorous stories: Antidote to despair?" *Gecko: A Journal of Deconstruction and Narrative Ideas in Therapeutic Practice* 2: 2–28.

Nasser, M. 1993. "A prescription of vomiting: Historical footnotes." *International Journal of Eating Disorders* 13(1): 129–131.

Needham, R. 1971. "Remarks on the analysis of kinship and marriage." In *Rethinking Kinship and Marriage*, ed. R. Needham. London: Tavistock.

New Idea. 1998. "Bronte's miracle cure." November 28, 14–17.

Nichter, M. 2008. "Coming to our senses: Appreciating the sensorial in medical anthropology." *Transcultural Psychiatry* 45: 163–197.

Nietsche, F. 1968. *The Will to Power*. Trans. and ed. W. Kaufman and R. J. Hollingdale. New York: Vintage Books.

Nuckolls, C. 1996. *The Cultural Dialectics of Knowledge and Desire*. Madison: University of Wisconsin Press.

Oakes-Ash, R. 2000. *Good Girls Do Swallow*. Melbourne: Random.

O'Connor, R. 2000. "Is anorexia a post-modern asceticism?" *Anthropology News*, February, 7–8.

O'Connor, R., and P. van Esterik. 2008. "Demedicalizing anorexia: A new cultural brokering." *Anthropology Today* 24(5): 6–9.

Olafson, F. 1987. *Heidegger and the Philosophy of Mind*. New Haven and London: Yale University Press.

Oliver, K., ed. 1993. *Ethics, Politics, and Difference in Julia Kristeva's Writing*. New York: Routledge.

Onions, C. T. 1966. *Oxford Dictionary of English Etymology*. Oxford: Clarendon Press.

Orbach, S. 1978. *Fat Is a Feminist Issue*. London: Hamlyn.

——. 1986. *Hunger Strike: The Anorectic's Struggle as a Metaphor for Our Age*. London: Faber and Faber.

Ortner, S. 1984. "Theory in anthropology since the sixties." *Comparative Studies in Society and History* 26(1): 126–166.

——. 1999. "Generation X anthropology in a media-saturated world." In *Critical Anthropology Now*, ed. G. Marcus, 55–87. Santa Fe, N.M.: School of American Research Press.

Ostrow, J. 1981. "Culture as a fundamental dimension of experience: A discussion of Pierre Bourdieu's theory of human habitus." *Human Studies* 4: 279–297.

Ottenberg, S. 1990. "Thirty years of fieldnotes: Changing relationships to the text." In *Fieldnotes: The Making of Anthropology*, ed. R. Sanjek, 139–160. Ithaca and London: Cornell University Press.

Parkin, R., and J. Eagles. 1993. "Blood-letting in bulimia nervosa." *British Journal of Psychiatry* 162: 246–248.

Parr, H., and C. Philo. 1995. "Mapping mad identities." In *Mapping the Subject: Geographies of Cultural Transformation*, ed. S. Pile and N. Thrift, 182–207. London: Routledge.

Peirano, M. 1998. "When anthropology is at home: The different contexts of a single discipline." *Annual Review of Anthropology* 27: 105–128.

Pembroke, L., ed. 1993. *Eating Distress: Perspectives from Personal Experience*. Chesham: Survivors Speak Out.

Perrot, P. 1984. *Les Dessus et les Dessous de la Bourgeoisie: Une Histoire du Vetement au XIXe siecle*. Bruxelles: Ed. Complexe.

Peters, N. 1987. "Close to the bone: Reviewing and redefining anorexia nervosa—a feminist perspective." Honours thesis, University of Western Australia.

———. 1995. "The ascetic anorexic." *Social Analysis* 37: 44–67.

Pike, K., and A. Borovoy. 2004. "The rise of eating disorders in Japan: Issues of culture and limitations of the model of 'westernization.'" *Culture, Medicine and Psychiatry* 28(4): 493–531.

Pizanias, C. 2000. "Habitus revisited: Notes and queries from the field." In *Pierre Bourdieu, Fieldwork in Culture*, ed. N. Brown and I. Szeman, 145–164. New York: Rowman and Littlefield.

Place, F. 1989. *Cardboard Lives*. Sydney: Local Consumption Publications.

Pope, H., and J. Hudson. 1992. "Is childhood sexual abuse a risk factor for bulimia nervosa?" *American Journal of Psychiatry* 149: 455–463.

Probyn, E. 1987. "The anorexic body." In *Body Invaders, Panic Sex in America*, ed. A. Kroker and M. Kroker, 199–211. New World Perspectives, CultureTexts Series. Montreal: Oxford University Press.

———. 1993. *Sexing the Self: Gendered Positions in Cultural Studies*. London and New York: Routledge.

———. 1996. *Outside Belongings*. London: Routledge.

———. 1999. "Beyond food/sex: Eating and an ethics of existence." *Theory, Culture and Society* 16(2): 215–228.

———. 2000. *Carnal Appetites: Food, Sex, Identities*. London and New York: Routledge.

Rabinow, P. 1977. *Reflections on Fieldwork in Morocco*. Berkeley: University of California Press.

Rampling, D. 1985. "Ascetic ideals and anorexia nervosa." *Journal of Psychiatric Research* 19(2/3): 89–94.

Rapport, N. 2000. "The narrative as fieldwork technique: Processual ethnography for a world in motion." In *Constructing the Field: Ethnographic Fieldwork in the Contemporary World*, ed. V. Amit, 71–95. London: Routledge.

Reineke, M. 1997. *Sacrificed Lives: Kristeva on Women and Violence*. Bloomington: Indiana University Press.

Rich, E. 2006. "Anorexic dis(connection): Managing anorexia as an illness and an identity." *Sociology of Health and Illness* 28(3): 284–305.

Robertson, M. 1992. *Starving in the Silences: An Exploration of Anorexia Nervosa*. Sydney: Allen and Unwin.

Roseman, M. 1991. *Healing Sounds from the Malaysian Rainforest: Temiar Music and Medicine*. Berkeley: University of California Press.

Rouse, R. 1991. "Mexican migration and the social space of postmodernity." *Diaspora* 1: 8–23.

Rozin, P., L. Millman, and C. Nemeroff. 1986. "Operation of the laws of sympathetic magic in disgust and other domains." *Journal of Personality and Social Psychology* 50(4): 703–712.

Russell, C., and P. Keel. 2002. "Homosexuality as a specific risk factor for eating disorders in men." *International Journal of Eating Disorders* 31(3): 300–306.

Sahlins, M. 1972. *Stone Age Economics*. Chicago: Aldine.

Sallis, E. 1998. *Hiam*. St. Leonards, N.S.W.: Allen and Unwin.

Sanjek, R. 1990. "A vocabulary for fieldnotes." In *Fieldnotes: The Making of Anthropology*, ed. R. Sanjek, 92–138. Ithaca and London: Cornell University Press.

Santich, B. 1995. *What the Doctors Ordered: 150 Years of Dietary Advice in Australia*. South Melbourne: Hyland House.

Saris, J. 1995. "Telling stories: Life histories, illness narratives, and institutional landscapes." *Culture, Medicine and Psychiatry* 19(1): 39–72.

Sass, L. 1992. "Heidegger, schizophrenia and the ontological difference." *Philosophical Psychology* 5(2): 109–132.

Schneider, D. 1980. *American Kinship: A Cultural Account*. 2nd. ed. Chicago: University of Chicago Press. First published 1968.

———. 1984. *A Critique of the Study of Kinship*. Ann Arbor: University of Michigan Press.

Seremetakis, N., ed. 1994. *The Senses Still: Perception and Memory as Material Culture in Modernity*. Boulder: Westview Press.

Serpell, L., J. Treasure, J. Teasdale, and V. Sullivan. 1999. "Anorexia nervosa: Friend or foe?" *International Journal of Eating Disorders* 25: 177–186.

Shildrick, M. 1997. *Leaky Bodies and Boundaries: Feminism, Postmodernism and (Bio)ethics*. London and New York: Routledge.

Shilling, C. 1991. "Educating the body: Physical capital and the production of social inequalities." *Sociology* 25(4): 653–672.

———. 1993. *The Body and Social Theory*. London: Sage.

Shils, E. 1956. *The Torment of Secrecy*. New York: Free Press.

Shullem, B. 1988. "The introduction of humor in supervision and therapy—Work is depressing enough without being too serious." *Journal of Strategic and Systemic Therapies* 7(2): 49–58.

Shute, J. 1992. *Life-Size*. Boston: Houghton Mifflin.

Sibley, D. 1995. *Geographies of Exclusion*. London and New York: Routledge.

Simmel, G. 1950. *The Sociology of George Simmel*. New York: Academic Press.

Smith, A. M. 1998. *Julia Kristeva: Speaking the Unspeakable*. London: Pluto Press.

Soja, E. 1995. "Heterotopologies: A remembrance of other spaces in the citadel-LA." In *Postmodern Cities and Spaces*, ed. S. Watson and K. Gibson, 13–34. Oxford: Blackwell.

Solomon, R. 1984. "Getting angry: The Jamesian theory of emotion in anthropology." In *Culture Theory: Essays on Mind, Self, and Emotion*, ed. R. Schweder and R. Levine, 238–254. Cambridge: Cambridge University Press.

Sorokin, P. 1941. *Man and Society in Calamity*. New York: Dutton.

Soros, E. 1998. "Giving death." *Differences* 10(1): 1–30.

Sours, J. 1980. *Starving to Death in a Sea of Objects*. New York: Aronson.

Spivak, G. 1981. "French feminism in an international frame." *Yale French Studies* 62: 154–184.

Stafford, C. 2000. "Chinese patriliny and the cycles of yang and laiwang." In *Cultures of Relatedness: New Approaches to the Study of Kinship*, ed. J. Carsten, 37–54. Cambridge: Cambridge University Press.

Stedman, T. 1995. *Stedman's Medical Dictionary. 26th ed.* Baltimore: Williams and Wilkins.

Steinhausen, H. 2002. "The outcome of anorexia nervosa in the 20th century." *American Journal of Psychiatry* 159: 1284–1293.

Stoller, P. 1989. *The Taste of Ethnographic Things: The Senses in Anthropology*. Philadelphia: University of Pennsylvania Press.

——. 1997. *Sensuous Scholarship*. Philadelphia: University of Pennsylvania Press.

Strathern, A. 1996. *Body Thoughts*. Ann Arbor: University of Michigan Press.

Strathern, M. 1988. *The Gender of the Gift*. Berkeley: University of California Press.

——. 1991. *Partial Connections*. Savage, Md.: Rowman and Littlefield.

——. 1992. *After Nature*. Cambridge: Cambridge University Press.

Strober, M. 2005. "The future of treatment research in anorexia nervosa." *International Journal of Eating Disorders* 37: 90–94.

Swartz, D. 1997. *Culture and Power: The Sociology of Pierre Bourdieu*. Chicago and London: University of Chicago Press.

Sykes, D. K., M. Gross, and S. Subishin. 1986. "Preliminary findings of demographic variables in patients suffering from anorexia nervosa and bulimia." *International Journal of Psychosomatics* 33(4): 27–30.

Szekely, E. 1988. *Never Too Thin*. Toronto: Women's Press.

Tait, G. 1992. "Anorexia nervosa: asceticism, differentiation, government." *Australian and New Zealand Journal of Sociology* 29(2): 194–208.

Tanzer, K. 1997. "When the 'I' means 'we.'" *Gecko: A Journal of Deconstruction and Narrative Ideas on Therapeutic Practice* 2: 65–77.

Taussig, M. 1980. "Reification and the consciousness of the patient." *Social Science and Medicine* 14: 3–13.

——. 1993. *Mimesis and Alterity: A Particular History of the Senses*. London: Routledge.

——. 1999. *Defacement: Public Secrecy and the Labor of the Negative*. Stanford, Calif.: Stanford University Press.

Telfer, J. 1998. *Per Alienus, Per Intimus: Agency and the Dialectics of Identity in Adoption*. PhD thesis, Department of Anthropology, Adelaide University.

Thomas, K. 1994. "Cleanliness and godliness in early modern England." In *Religion, Culture and Society in Early Modern Britain*, ed. A. Fletcher and P. Roberts, 56–83. Cambridge: Cambridge University Press.

Thomas, M. 1999. *Dreams in the Shadows: Vietnamese-Australian Lives in Transition*. Sydney: Allen and Unwin.

Thornton, C., and J. Russell. 1997. "Obsessive compulsive comorbidity in the dieting disorders." *International Journal of Eating Disorders* 21(1): 83–87.

Throop, J. 2005. "Hypocognition, a "sense of the uncanny," and the anthropology of ambiguity: Reflections on Robert I. Levy's contribution to theories of experience in anthropology." *Ethos* 33(4): 499–511.

Throop, J., and K. Murphy. 2002. "Bourdieu and phenomenology: A critical assessment." *Anthropological Theory* 2(2): 185–207.

Tomso, G. 2004. "Bug chasing, barebacking and the risks of care." *Literature and Medicine* 23(1): 88–111.

Torgovnick, M. 1990. *Gone Primitive: Savage Intellectuals, Modern Lives*. Chicago: University of Chicago Press.

Tsing, A. 1993. *In the Realm of the Diamond Queen*. Princeton: Princeton University Press.

Turner, B. 1982. "The government of the body: Medical regimens and the rationalization of diet." *British Journal of Sociology* 33(2): 254–269.

——. 1984. *The Body and Society: Explorations in Social Theory*. London: Blackwell.

——. 1987. *Medical Power and Social Knowledge*. London: Sage.

Turner, V. 1970. *The Forest of Symbols*. Ithaca: Cornell University Press.

Ussher, J. 1991. *Women's Madness: Misogyny or Mental Illness?* London: Harvester Wheatsheaf.

Vandereycken, W. 1993. "Blood-letting in bulimia nervosa." *British Journal of Psychiatry* 162: 851.

Vandereycken, W., and R. van Deth. 1994. *From Fasting Saints to Anorexic Girls: The History of Self-Starvation.* New York: New York University Press.

Vertinsky, P. 1994. *The Eternally Wounded Woman.* Manchester: Illini Books.

Vice, S. 1997. *Introducing Bakhtin.* Manchester: Manchester University Press.

Vigarello, G. 1988. *Concepts of Cleanliness: Changing Attitudes in France Since the Middle Ages.* Cambridge: Cambridge University Press.

Visser, M. 1992. *The Rituals of Dinner.* New York: Penguin.

Wafer, J. 1996. "After the field." In *Things As They Are: New Directions in Phenomenological Anthropology*, ed. M. Jackson, 259–272. Bloomington and Indianapolis: Indiana University Press.

Waller, G., C. Halek, and A. Crisp. 1993. "Sexual abuse as a factor in anorexia nervosa: Evidence from two separate case series." *Journal of Psychosomatic Research* 37(8): 873–879.

Warin, M. 2000. "The glass cage: An ethnography of exposure in schizophrenia." *Health: An Interdisciplinary Journal for the Social Study of Health, Illness and Medicine* 4(1): 115–133.

———. 2005. "Transformations of intimacy and sociality: Bedrooms in public institutions." *Body and Society* 11(3): 97–113.

Weber, M. 1930. *The Protestant Ethic and the Spirit of Capitalism.* London: Unwin University Books.

Wedgewood, C. 1930. "The Nature and Function of Secrets." *Oceania* 1: 130–145.

Weedon, C. 1987. *Feminist Practice and Poststructuralist Theory.* Oxford: Blackwell.

Weltzin, E., N. Weisensel, D. Franczyk, K. Burnett, C. Klitz, and P. Bean. 2005. "Eating disorders in men: Update." *Journal of Men's Health and Gender* 2(2): 186–193.

Weiner, A. 1976. *Women of Value, Men of Renown.* Austin: University of Texas Press.

Weiner, J. 1995. "Anthropologists, historians and the secret of social knowledge." *Anthropology Today* 11(5): 3–7.

White, M., and D. Epston. 1989. *Literate Means to Therapeutic Ends.* Adelaide: Dulwich Center.

Wolf, M. 1992. *A Thrice Told Tale.* Stanford, Calif.: Stanford University Press.

Wolf, N. 1990. *The Beauty Myth.* London: Vintage Books.

Women's Health Project. 1992. *Living with the Culture of Control.* Queensland: National Better Health Program.

Wood, C. 1981. "The doctors' dilemma; Sin, salvation and the menstrual cycle in medieval thought." *Speculum* 56: 710–727.

Wood, P. 1997. "Body boundaries: Using the metaphor of body in understanding public health practice in nineteenth century Dunedin." In *Bodily Boundaries, Sexualized Genders and Medical Discourses*, ed. M. de Ras and V. Grace, 27–38. Palmerston North: Dunmore Press.

World Health Organization. 1992. *ICD-10: Classification of Mental and Behavioral Disorders: Clinical Descriptions and Diagnostic Guidelines.* Geneva: World Health Organization.

Yao, S. 1993. "A room named desire: Body, space and the bathroom in the Australian home." *Broadsheet* 22(1): 3–7.

Yep, G., K. Lovaas, and A. Pagonis. 2002. "The case of 'riding bareback': Sexual practices and the paradoxes of identity in the era of AIDS." *Journal of Homosexuality* 42(4): 1–14.

Young, M. 1983. *Magicians of Manumanua: Living Myth in Kalauna.* Berkeley: University of California Press.

Zerbe, K. 1993. *The Body Betrayed: A Deeper Understanding of Women, Eating Disorders and Treatment*. Carlsbad, Calif.: Gurze Books.

Zipfel, S., B. Lowe, D. Reas, H. Deter, and W. Herzog. 2000. "Long-term prognosis in anorexia nervosa: Lessons from a 21-year follow-up study." *Lancet* 355: 721–722.

Zubieta, J., M. Demitrack, A. Fenick, and D. Krahn. 1995. "Obsessionality in eating disorder patients: Relationship to clinical presentation and two-year outcome." *Journal of Psychiatric Research* 29(4): 333–342.

INDEX

ABOUT THE AUTHOR

MEGAN WARIN is a social anthropologist whose research focuses on phenomenological approaches to gendered bodies, memory and migration among Persian women, and cultural psychiatry. Warin has taught in a number of academic institutions, including the University of Adelaide and Flinders University of South Australia in Australia, and Durham University in the United Kingdom.